PENGUIN BOOKS

the CSIRO healthy heart program

Associate Professor Manny Noakes is the stream leader for the Diet and Lifestyle program at CSIRO Human Nutrition, a multidisciplinary team of nutritionists, psychologists and exercise physiologists engaged in developing innovative programs for improving healthy lifestyle behaviour among Australians. She also ma   es clinical trials that provide scientific evidence for the efficacy of diet and exercise programs   lth. Manny has published over 100 scientific papers, with a major emphasis on diet comp   weight-loss and cardiovascular health. She is a senior lecturer in the School of Medicine, F' c niversity, affiliate senior lecturer in the Department of Obstetrics and Gynaecology, Universi   laide, and affiliate associate professor in the Department of Medicine, University of Adelaide

Professor Peter C   the scientific director for clinical nutrition, obesity and related conditions at CSIRO Human   on. He is also professor of medicine at the University of Adelaide, and practises as an endocrir   at the Royal Adelaide Hospital and the Flinders Medical Centre. Peter is a frequent and sough   speaker at national and international conferences and is also widely published in the areas   functional foods and heart health. His personal research interests are in the areas of diet, obe   diovascular disease, and optimal diets for people with insulin resistance and diabetes.

The Commonwea t   ientific and Industrial Research Organisation (CSIRO), Australia's national science agency   een dedicated to the practical application of knowledge and science for society and industry   1928, and today ranks in the top one per cent of world scientific institutions in 12 of 22 rese   elds. CSIRO Human Nutrition conducts research into human health, including disease prev   diagnosis and innovative treatment. CSIRO Human Nutrition is a centre of Food Scien   , a joint venture between CSIRO and the Victorian Government that is Australia's largest   diversified food research organisation.

D0582652

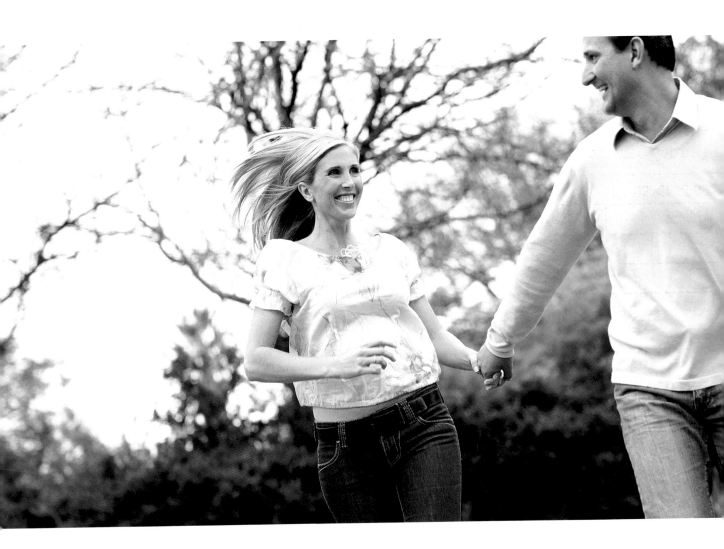

the CSIRO healthy heart program

dr manny noakes
& dr peter clifton

CSIRO

PENGUIN BOOKS

Published by the Penguin Group
Penguin Group (Australia)
250 Camberwell Road, Camberwell, Victoria 3124, Australia
(a division of Pearson Australia Group Pty Ltd)
Penguin Group (USA) Inc
375 Hudson Street, New York, New York 10014, USA
Penguin Group (Canada)
90 Eglinton Avenue East, Suite 700, Toronto, Canada ON M4P 2Y3
(a division of Pearson Penguin Canada Inc.)
Penguin Books Ltd
80 Strand, London WC2R 0RL England
Penguin Ireland
25 St Stephen's Green, Dublin 2, Ireland
(a division of Penguin Books Ltd)
Penguin Books India Pvt Ltd
11 Community Centre, Panchsheel Park, New Delhi – 110 017, India
Penguin Group (NZ)
67 Apollo Drive, Rosedale, North Shore 0632, New Zealand
(a division of Pearson New Zealand Ltd)
Penguin Books (South Africa) (Pty) Ltd
24 Sturdee Avenue, Rosebank, Johannesburg 2196, South Africa

Penguin Books Ltd, Registered Offices: 80 Strand, London, WC2R 0RL, England

First published by Penguin Group (Australia), 2008

10 9 8 7 6 5 4 3 2 1

Text copyright © CSIRO 2008

The following brand names used in this book are registered trade marks of the following companies: Equal (p 245) – Merisant; Flora pro-activ (pp 99, 112) – Unilever; Guinness (pp 212, 213, 268, 269) – Guinness & Co.; Kellog's Guardian (pp 124, 137, 129, 131, 133, 137, 139, 141, 143, 145, 149, 266) – Kellogg (Aust.) Pty Ltd; Logicol (pp 99, 112) – Goodman Fielder Consumer Foods Pty Ltd; Mountain Bread (pp 106, 127, 147, 267, 270) – Mountain Bread Pty Ltd; Nuttelex Pulse (p 99) – Nuttelex Pty Ltd; Sanitarium Vegie Delights (pp 158, 208, 268, 270, 271) – Sanitarium Health Food Company; Tabasco (pp 206, 250, 266) – McIlhenny Company; Uncle Tobys Healthwise (pp 124, 127, 129, 131, 133, 135, 137, 139, 141, 143, 145, 147, 149, 266) and Uncle Tobys Oatbrits (pp 124, 127, 133, 135, 137, 139, 143, 147, 149, 266) – Société des Produits Nestle SA; Yoplait Heart Active (p 99) and Pura Heart Active (pp 99, 112) – National Foods.

The moral right of the authors has been asserted

Design by Nikki Townsend and Megan Baker © Penguin Group (Australia)
Photographs on pp vii (middle), 152–65, 169–71, 177–97, 200–201, 207–35 and 241–49 by Ian Wallace; on pp vi (left & middle), vii (left & right), 1–6, 14–24, 28, 33–42, 54, 59–72, 77–93, 100, 103–108, 114–18, 121, 134–36, 142, 166, 252–71 by Nicholas Wilson; pp 120 by Jupiter Images; all other images by Getty Images
Food styling by Louise Pickford
Food preparation by Jennifer Tolhurst
Recipes by Heidi Flett
Typeset in 10.75/16.5 Berkeley Oldstyle Book by Post Pre-press Group, Brisbane, Queensland
Colour reproduction by Splitting Image, Clayton, Victoria
Printed and bound in China by Everbest Printing Co. Ltd

National Library of Australia
Cataloguing-in-Publication data:

Noakes, Manny (Manila), 1953–
The CSIRO healthy heart program / Manny Noakes, Peter Clifton.
9780143009047 (pbk)
Includes index.
Cardiovascular system – Diseases – Nutritional aspects.
Cardiovascular system – Diseases – Prevention.
Clifton, Peter M. CSIRO.

616.10654

Contents

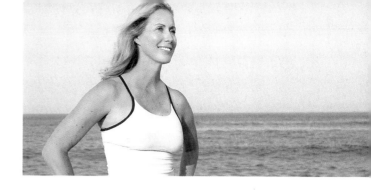

Dedication	vi
Acknowledgements	vii
Introduction	**1**
Part 1 Cardiovascular health stocktake	**7**
Ten warning signs of poor heart health	9
1 Family history	9
2 High blood cholesterol and triglycerides and low HDL	9
3 Excess weight	10
4 High blood pressure	11
5 High blood glucose	12
6 Lack of exercise	12
7 Smoking	12
8 Sleep apnoea	12
9 Depressed mood	13
10 Sexual problems	13
Part 2 Body, heart and mind	**15**
Weight and waistline	17
Cholesterol levels	22
Blood pressure	27
Blood glucose and type 2 diabetes	31
Exercise for a healthy heart	34
Sex matters	39
Depression and dealing with stress	42
Sleep apnoea and a good night's sleep	49
Motivation – mind over matter	51
Part 3 The CLIP exercise program	**57**
First things first	59
Warm-up, stretch and cool-down	61
Stretching exercises	62
Walking program	68
Muscle-strengthening program	73
Part 4 Ten super CLIP foods	**91**
Good food for good health	93
1 Fish and omega-3 fatty acids	93
2 Soluble fibre	95
3 Low-fat dairy foods	95
4 Nuts	96
5 Legumes	96
6 Whole grains	97
7 Alcohol	98
8 Plant sterols	98
9 Lean protein foods	99
10 Oils and seeds	99
Part 5 CLIP and you	**101**
What is the CLIP eating plan?	103
Your daily food allowance on the CLIP basic plan	106
Choosing your kilojoule level for CLIP	108
Vegetarians and CLIP	110
Eating out on CLIP	113
The CLIP eating plan: frequently asked questions	115
The CLIP weight and cholesterol maintenance plan	120
Part 6 CLIP menu plans	**123**
Part 7 CLIP recipes	**151**
Glossary	252
Appendices	255
Index	272

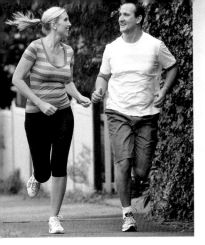
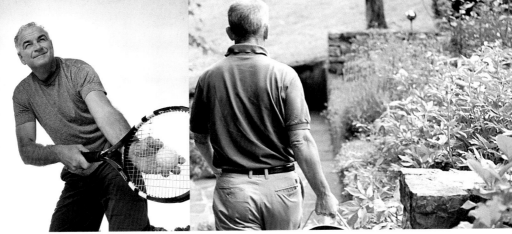

Dedication

This book is dedicated to Professor Paul Nestel AO, MD, FRACP, FTSE, FCSANZ, who established the CSIRO Clinical Research Unit in Adelaide in 1986 as a bicentennial project of the Heart Foundation. Paul is an international authority on the cause and management of diseases of the arteries and has published over 420 scientific and medical papers. He is also an Officer of the Order of Australia and a former chief of CSIRO Human Nutrition. Paul is an active and young 79-year-old who continues his work as a senior academic staff member at the Baker Heart Research Institute and is an Honorary Professor of Medicine at Deakin University.

Paul's vision was 'to develop a diet for Australians that is optimal with respect to known risk factors for cardiovascular disease, and is at the same time practical, acceptable and safe'. We hope we have gone a long way to realising that goal with this publication, which is the culmination of much of the research Paul initiated and conducted at CSIRO.

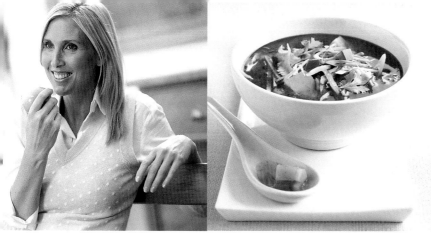
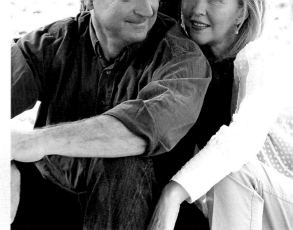

Acknowledgements

We would like to acknowledge the following people who painstakingly reviewed our manuscript. Their invaluable feedback has assisted us in improving the readability, accuracy and emphasis for our readers:

- Professor Paul Nestel AO, MD, FRACP, FTSE, FCSANZ
- Dr David Sullivan, physician and pathologist, FRACP, FRCPA
- Barbara Eden, Food Supply Policy Manager, Heart Foundation
- Dr Peter Abernethy, National Director of Cardiovascular Health Programs, Heart Foundation

The messages in this book concur with the health messages from the National Heart Foundation of Australia. The Heart Foundation saves lives and improves health through funding world-class cardiovascular research, guidelines for health professionals, informing the public and assisting people with cardiovascular disease. As a charity, the Heart Foundation relies on donations and gifts in wills to continue its life-saving research, education and health-promotion work. For further information on heart health visit www.heartfoundation.org.au or call 1300 36 27 87.

Finally, we would like to thank Nicola Young, Nikki Townsend, Megan Baker, Sue Van Velsen, Ingrid Ohlsson and Julie Gibbs of Penguin for their endless patience and hard work in taking this publication from manuscript to masterpiece.

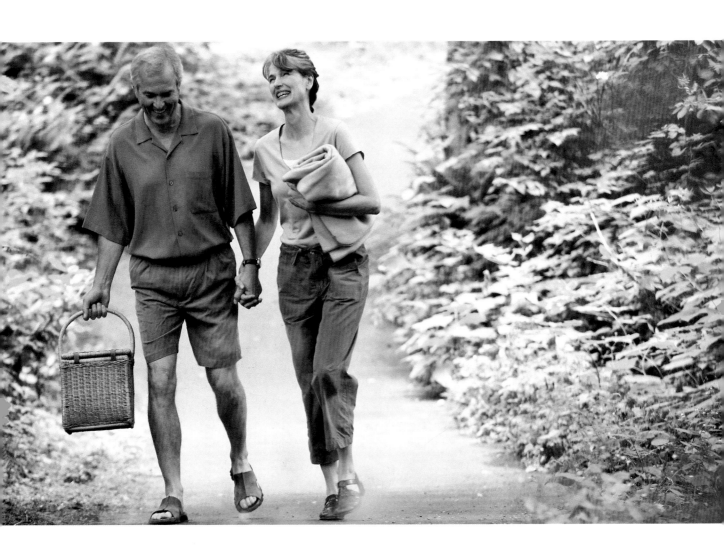

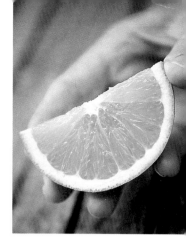

Introduction

As we age, we start to take our health more seriously, so that we can keep enjoying life for as long as possible. Although it is best to start living healthily in childhood, it is never too late to start.

This book is aimed at helping you understand some of the key health issues that can arise when we are in our 40s and beyond. It will show you how to maintain a healthy diet and exercise program for overall wellbeing. Above all, it will help you stay in control of your health so that you can enjoy life to the full.

This book's focus is on keeping your heart and blood vessels healthy; we call this our cardiovascular health. You might think that 'heart disease' is just that, but in reality the root causes of heart disease are problems with our arteries, blood pressure and circulation, rather than our heart alone. A more appropriate term, therefore, and the one we'll be using throughout this book, is cardiovascular disease (CVD). Generally, the diet and lifestyle approach that best takes care of our circulatory system also provides the nutrition our bodies need to function at their best as we age. It can also help lower our risk of other chronic diseases, such as osteoporosis, osteoarthritis and cancer.

In our adolescence, our arteries begin to lay down fatty deposits containing cholesterol, usually as a result of our poor diet and lifestyle choices. The body responds to this by triggering inflammation. Even at a low level, this inflammation can, over time, do permanent damage to the elasticity of our arteries. Along with an accumulation of cholesterol in a wide variety of cells, this can cause our arteries to narrow. This is called atherosclerosis and it can be accelerated if you have other risk factors such as high blood cholesterol, high blood pressure or if you smoke. Atherosclerosis can result in many conditions, including angina (heart pain on exertion).

Our circulatory system is extremely important in maintaining our health. It uses blood pumped by our heart to carry nutrients, water, oxygen and waste products to and from our body cells. The blood does this by travelling through blood vessels, which are found throughout the body. Arteries are blood vessels that carry blood away from the heart. The narrowing of our arteries as a result of our diet and lifestyle impacts on the way blood is delivered throughout our body. When the arteries that circulate blood to the legs and feet are affected, common symptoms include cramping, numbness or fatigue, particularly in the legs and buttocks during exercise. Less well known is that damage to the blood vessels to and within the brain can also occur. In men, atherosclerosis can also affect the blood vessels in the penis, making it difficult to sustain an erection. More seriously, if the fatty deposits in the artery walls become unstable, this can result in a clot, which could lead to a heart attack or stroke.

Our previous publications, *The CSIRO Total Well-being Diet* books 1 and 2, provided a good foundation for a healthy diet and lifestyle and for managing your weight. They are also well suited for achieving cardiovascular health, and will complement the lifestyle approach in this book. *The CSIRO Healthy Heart Program* will provide you with more options in eating styles and maximise the benefits for your cardiovascular health.

Although your susceptibility to atherosclerosis and its causative risk factors such as high blood pressure will be partly determined by your genetic make-up and your age, you can make many changes to your diet and lifestyle that will help. We all have deposits on our arteries, even in our youth, and they build up as we age. The good news is that we can delay their build-up with a healthy lifestyle, and the earlier we start the better. There is even evidence that it is possible to reverse this damage partially by making lifestyle changes and using medication. The lifestyle factors that can make a difference are:

- maintaining a healthy diet
- not smoking
- keeping your blood cholesterol low
- doing regular exercise
- losing weight if you are overweight or obese
- lowering your blood pressure to normal, and
- preventing type 2 diabetes or keeping it in check with weight control and exercise.

To help you make and maintain these changes to your lifestyle, we at CSIRO have developed a comprehensive diet and exercise program we call CLIP, the **C**omplete **LI**festyle **P**rogram.

Are you at high risk of heart attack or stroke?

You are at high risk of heart attack or stroke if you answer yes to any of the following questions.

- Are you overweight with high triglyceride levels, low HDL ('good') cholesterol levels, high blood pressure or glucose intolerance?
- Do you have diabetes? If you have type 2 diabetes and an LDL ('bad') cholesterol level of 2.5 mmol/L or more (see page 265), you are at increased risk of developing CVD.
- Do you have chronic kidney disease?
- Have you been diagnosed with familial hypercholesterolaemia (see page 23)?
- Do you have an Aboriginal or Torres Strait Islander background?
- Do you have a family history of premature heart disease? That is, a first-degree relative who had heart disease before the age of 60?

CLIP (the Complete LIfestyle Program)

Although it is important to keep your blood cholesterol low, this is not the only consideration when devising a diet for healthy arteries. We know that many foods contain components that can help – such as good fats from fish and nuts, and soluble fibre from oats, wholegrain cereals, fruit and vegetables. Many large-scale studies have shown that people who eat high levels of these foods have lower rates of heart disease.

To help you through the maze of lifestyle advice to changes that work, our team of scientists has created CLIP. Our trials have shown that CLIP can lower blood cholesterol by an average of 15–20 per cent and reduce weight on average by 4.5 kilograms in six weeks and 9 kilograms over 12 weeks. CLIP can also decrease blood pressure and artery inflammation, and reduce triglyceride levels (triglycerides are blood fats indicative of heart-disease risk) by 15 per cent.

But we devised the CLIP eating plan not only to provide these great health benefits, but also because it's full of tasty foods you'll love.

CLIP and weight loss

The CLIP eating plan was originally created for people who needed to lose weight. However, we have now adapted the program so that it is suitable for anyone who wants to improve their lifestyle and cardiovascular health. It is aimed in particular at people with high cholesterol and/or blood pressure. If you do not need to lose weight but still have high cholesterol, you can easily modify this eating plan to suit your needs.

Our CLIP study

Since the early 1990s, we at CSIRO Human Nutrition have performed many clinical trials around nutrition and exercise. In more recent years, we have also researched concentrated food components that can reduce blood cholesterol levels. Today, these food components, such as plant extracts called sterols, are available in what we call 'functional foods'.

In our CLIP trial, one group of our volunteers followed CLIP for six weeks, another group followed more general lifestyle advice, and a third followed this same general advice *and* took a low dose of statins, drugs commonly used to lower cholesterol (see page 26).

The people in the group that combined general lifestyle advice with statins experienced the greatest reduction in LDL (bad) cholesterol and triglycerides. However, the people in this group did not lose as much weight or lose as much fat from their waistlines as those following the CLIP eating plan. This indicates that, for this group, the majority of the reduction in LDL cholesterol and triglycerides was due to the use of a prescription medication – and we all want to avoid those for as long as we possibly can.

By following a healthy lifestyle program such as CLIP, you may be able to avoid or delay the need for blood-cholesterol-lowering medications. If you are already taking such medication, CLIP is an ideal way to improve your health.

About this book

This book is divided into seven sections. In **Part 1** we look at the ten main warning signs of cardiovascular disease and provide you with basic tools to assess which of these warning signs apply to you. In **Part 2** we explain these in more detail and look at some other key areas relevant to cardiovascular health, including tips on maintaining a healthy lifestyle. In **Part 3** we offer advice on getting active, including a 12-week exercise plan that complements the eating plan and takes care of both your aerobic and strength-training needs. In **Part 4** we examine the ten key nutrient components of the CLIP eating plan and explain why they are so good for you.

This is followed by **Part 5**, in which we explain CLIP in greater detail. There you will find more information on the key foods in the plan and what you need to eat each day. We have also tried to answer all your questions in our 'Frequently asked questions' section. But making a lifestyle change is only half the challenge – the other half is maintaining it. To help you with this we have developed a comprehensive maintenance approach that includes tips and hints for staying healthy.

In **Part 6** we provide two six-week menu plans based on the CLIP eating plan, while **Part 7** offers an array of delicious recipes to get you started with CLIP.

Good luck, and good health.

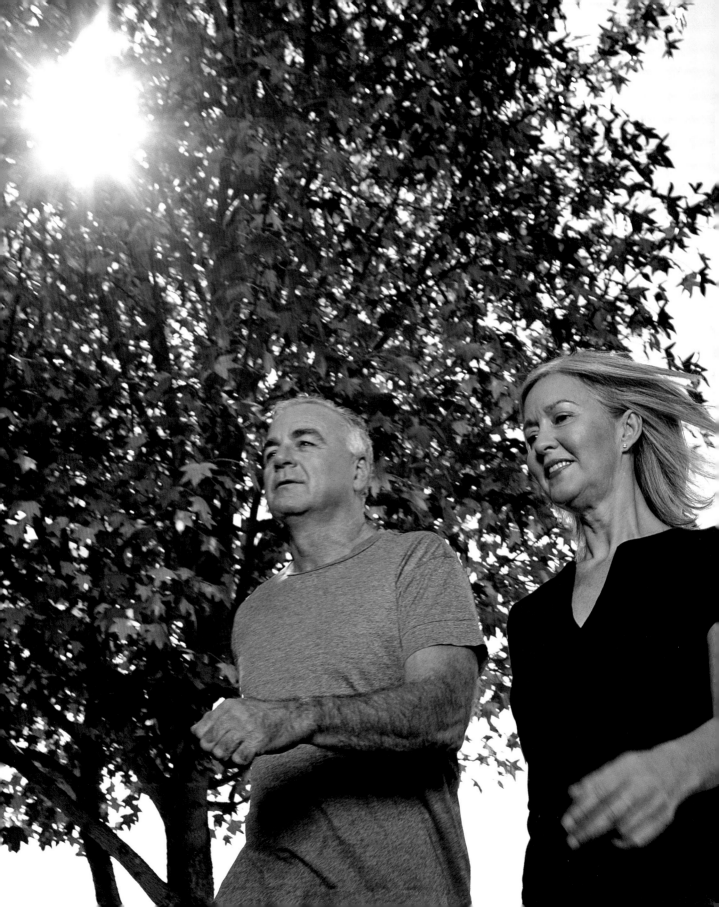

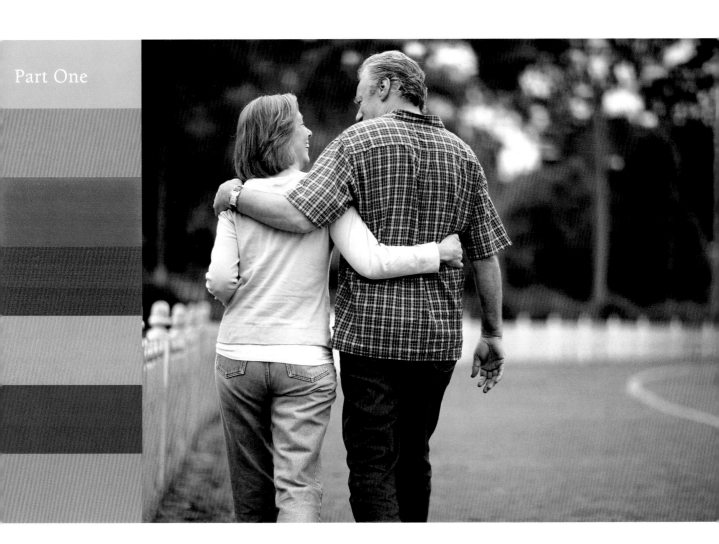

Part One

Cardiovascular health stocktake

by Dr Manny Noakes, Dr Peter Clifton, Dr Grant Brinkworth,
Dr Jennifer Keogh, Xenia Cleanthous, Lynn Field,
Adam Harrison, Dr Jane Bowen and Belinda Wyld

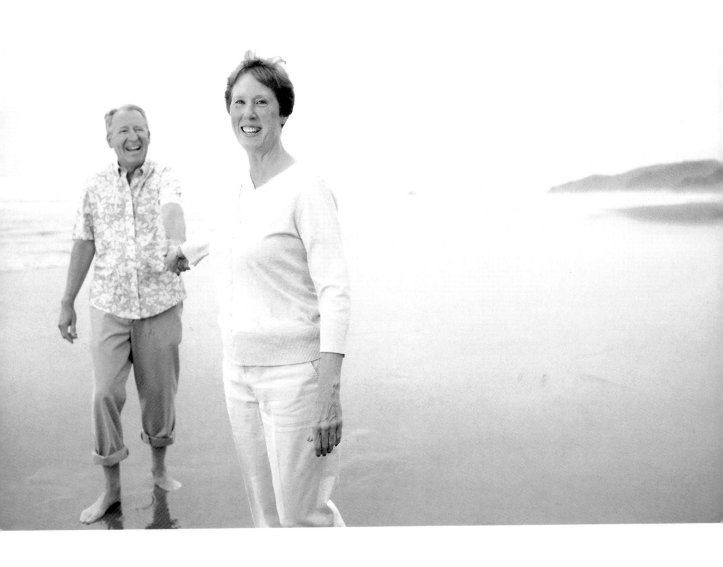

Ten warning signs of poor heart health

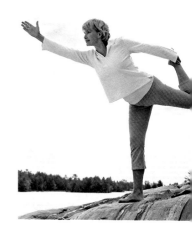

If you need motivation to improve your cardiovascular health, start by checking your vital statistics.

In spite of our rising obesity levels, 40 per cent of Australian men and 15 per cent of Australian women who carry excess weight think that their weight is normal. Start with a visit to your doctor for a check-up and blood test. Once you have all the results, make sure you keep a record of your measurements for the cardiovascular health indicators in the table on page 265. Check your measurements again after you have completed the first six weeks of CLIP. You will probably be amazed at the difference, and this will maintain your motivation. An annual check-up will then help you keep track of your progress.

The following pages indicate ten warning signs of cardiovascular disease (CVD) to watch out for in your quest for better cardiovascular health.

1   Family history

If one of your parents or a sibling developed CVD before the age of 60, you are at increased risk of developing CVD as well. Although you can't modify your genes,

you can still significantly reduce your risk by taking into account the risk factors we've already mentioned and doing your best to reduce them.

Familial hypercholesterolaemia is an inherited genetic disorder that can greatly increase the risk of heart attack. This condition calls for lifelong drug treatment in combination with a healthy lifestyle. See page 23 for more information.

2   High blood cholesterol and triglycerides and low HDL

Regular cholesterol checks can help you keep an eye on your cardiovascular health, especially if you are over the age of 45. The lab will measure your total cholesterol, high-density lipoprotein (HDL) cholesterol ('good' cholesterol), low-density lipoprotein (LDL) cholesterol ('bad' cholesterol), and HDL:LDL cholesterol ratio (cholesterol status). You should also receive a measurement of your blood triglyceride levels.

Once you know your current cholesterol and triglyceride levels, or if you know them already, compare them with values in the table on page 265. If you are already aware that you have heart and/or blood pressure problems, pay particular attention to the targets in the right-hand column. For more information on triglycerides and cholesterol, see page 22.

If you are not in a high-risk category, how low you should aim for your LDL cholesterol level will depend on your risk of developing CVD or having a heart attack in the future. The higher your risk, the more important it is to lower your LDL cholesterol levels and control any other CVD risk factors (including smoking and high blood pressure), and the more you will benefit from immediate action.

The New Zealand Heart Disease Risk Calculator (see - www.nzgg.org.nz/guidelines/0035/CVD_Risk_Chart.pdf) calculates your probability of developing heart disease in the next five years by using your age, blood pressure, diabetes status, smoking habits and the ratio of your total cholesterol to HDL cholesterol. A score of less than 10 per cent means a mild risk, whereas a score of greater than 30 per cent means you have a high risk. Your GP can use your score as a guide to whether you need medication to lower some of your risk factors.

3   Excess weight

There are three simple measures of whether you are overweight or obese: your weight, your body mass index (BMI) and your waist circumference. BMI and waist circumference combined give a good indication of your CVD risk.

BMI (body mass index)

BMI is calculated using your weight in kilograms and your height in metres.

$$BMI = \text{weight in kilograms}/(\text{height in metres})^2$$

example

Louisa is 57 years old, weighs 78 kilograms and is 158 centimetres (1.58 metres) tall. Her BMI is:

78 divided by 1.58 squared: $78/(1.58)^2 = 31.2$

Consulting the table below, we can see that Louisa's BMI indicates she is obese.

What your BMI tells you

BMI	body condition
less than 18.4	underweight
18.5–24.9	normal (target)
25–29.9	overweight
more than 30	obese

example

Martin is 50 years old, weighs 83 kilograms and is 180 centimetres (1.80 metres) tall. His BMI is:

83 divided by 1.80 squared: $83/(1.80)^2 = 25.6$

Martin's BMI indicates that he is slightly overweight.

Note that these BMI values apply only to adults aged 18 years and over, and are based on studies of Caucasian populations. This means that they are not applicable to children and adolescents and may not be appropriate for people of non-European backgrounds, particularly Asian, Aboriginal and Torres Strait Islander people. For instance, people with an Asian background generally carry less excess body fat and have lower BMIs than Caucasians. The same applies to waist-circumference measurements.

Waist circumference

Too much fat around your abdomen is also a risk factor for CVD, whatever your weight or BMI. Your abdominal fat can be measured in terms of your waist circumference. To measure your waist circumference, place the tape measure around your bare abdomen at the narrowest point between your ribs and hips. Ensure the tape is snug but does not push tightly into your skin. Measure your waist circumference after breathing out normally – do not 'suck in' your tummy. Read the tape measure and record your waist circumference in centimetres.

Waist circumference and health for Caucasians

	female waist circumference	male waist circumference
normal (target)	less than 80 cm	less than 94 cm
increased risk of health complications	80–88 cm	94–102 cm
substantially increased risk of health complications	more than 88 cm	more than 102 cm

These figures apply to south Asian and Chinese women, but Japanese women should aim for less than 75 centimetres. South Asian and Chinese men should aim for less than 90 centimetres, while for Japanese men this should be less than 85 centimetres.

Combined with your BMI, your waist circumference is a very good measure of your CVD risk. Consult the table below once you have calculated your BMI and measured your waist circumference.

4   High blood pressure

Blood pressure is the pressure generated by your heart as it pumps blood into the aorta (the largest blood vessel), which enables the blood to circulate to your toes and back. Blood pressure is usually measured using a device called a sphygmomanometer (pronounced sfigmo-manom-eter). A cuff is fitted around your upper arm and inflated to measure your blood pressure. Blood pressure values are recorded in millimetres of mercury (mmHg). The doctor or nurse who takes your blood pressure will give you two values – the systolic pressure and the diastolic pressure. Systolic pressure is the highest pressure during each heart beat and diastolic is the lowest.

High blood pressure can cause serious health problems such as heart attack, stroke or kidney disease. There are usually no warning symptoms, so it is important to have your blood pressure checked regularly.

Normal blood pressure is defined as less than $^{120}/_{80}$. A high to normal blood pressure is $^{120-139}/_{80-89}$. For more information on blood pressure see page 27.

BMI, waist circumference and CVD risk for Caucasians

body condition	BMI	waist circumference	
		80–88 cm (🧍) or 94–102 cm (🧍)	more than 88 cm (🧍) or 102 cm (🧍)
underweight	18.4 or less	—	—
target (normal)	18.5–24.9	—	increased risk
overweight	25–29.9	increased risk	high risk
obese	30 or more	high risk	very high risk

5   High blood glucose

To find out if you have type 2 diabetes or a related condition called pre-diabetes, your doctor will take a blood sample to find out your blood glucose levels. You may also be asked to take an oral glucose tolerance test (OGTT). For this test, you follow a high-carbohydrate diet for three days then fast for 12 hours. An initial blood sample is taken to check your fasting blood glucose levels. You are then given a glucose drink and have your blood taken 1 hour and 2 hours later. Normally, your body would be able to metabolise this glucose within 2 hours. If your doctor diagnoses either of the following two conditions, you do not have type 2 diabetes but you are at increased risk of developing it in the future.

1   IFG (impaired fasting glucose) – fasting blood glucose levels are higher than normal but do not rise abnormally after a glucose drink.
2   IGT (impaired glucose tolerance) – blood glucose levels after the glucose drink are higher than normal, but not high enough to diagnose diabetes.

For more information on blood glucose and type 2 diabetes, see page 31.

6   Lack of exercise

Lack of exercise is one of the main contributing lifestyle risk factors for atherosclerosis and CVD. Aim for at least 30 minutes of moderate-intensity physical activity on most, preferably all, days.

Before you begin any exercise program you should consult your doctor, especially if you have a medical condition or have not exercised for a while. If you are new to exercise, you need to start slowly. Look for opportunities to be active throughout the day and use the talk test on page 71 to gauge how hard you are working and monitor your increasing fitness level.

For more information on how to increase your activity levels, see page 34. See page 59 for our exercise plan, which is suitable whether you are new to exercise or are already reasonably physically active.

7   Smoking

The single most important thing you can do to reduce your risk of CVD is avoid smoking and second-hand smoke. Smoking can increase your risk of blood clots and 'harden' your artery walls.

People who smoke are at a 70 per cent greater risk of death from CVD than those who do not. After one year of no smoking, your risk will have been reduced by 50 per cent. After 15 years of no smoking, your risk will be about the same as that of people who have never smoked.

8   Sleep apnoea

While there are many reasons for poor quality of sleep, people often complain that snoring is a problem. Snoring can interrupt our sleep and cause daytime drowsiness or lethargy, but it can also be an indication that something is wrong. For many people, men in particular, snoring can be a symptom of a condition called sleep apnoea. Sleep apnoea results when excess body fat in the neck presses on the main tubes to the lungs. In deep sleep, the walls of the tubes are sucked together. This completely blocks the entry of air into the lungs and reduces the oxygen level in the blood. The sleeper doesn't usually wake up, but they tend to rouse slightly before drifting back to sleep almost immediately. Their quality of sleep is ruined.

The risks of untreated sleep apnoea include heart attack, stroke, impotence, irregular heartbeat, high blood pressure and CVD – all good reasons to seek treatment as soon as possible. Weight loss can alleviate the symptoms of sleep apnoea. See page 49 for more.

9   Depressed mood

People who experience depression, are socially isolated or do not have quality social support are at greater risk of developing CVD. These three factors can have as great an impact on our susceptibility to CVD as other, better known warning signs.

When we are depressed, support from our family and friends is vital if we are to heal, so when we are isolated or have a limited support network, stress can do long-term damage to our body. Here are some telltale signs that you may be depressed.

- Your sleep is disrupted or of poor quality, and you are especially susceptible to waking early in the morning.
- You are tense and irritable without good reason.
- You are worrying more than usual.
- You have difficulty concentrating.
- You feel tired for no reason.
- You are sometimes so nervous you can't calm down.
- You are sometimes so restless you can't sit still.
- You feel so sad you cannot cheer up.
- You experience frequent feelings of worthlessness and hopelessness.
- Everything seems to be an effort for you.

For more information on depression, and checklists for identifying depression and how to deal with it, visit www.beyondblue.org.au. And on page 42 we provide tips and information on managing stress, which is an important means of avoiding depression.

10 Sexual problems

While sexual problems are not in themselves a cause of vascular problems, they can be an early warning sign that you may be at risk of developing CVD. Many of the risk factors associated with CVD can also affect your sex drive and ability to enjoy a sexual relationship. Sexual health is dependent on many factors, including hormone levels, blood flow and the health of the nervous system. Some men who carry excess weight and have high blood pressure can experience erectile dysfunction, and weight loss can often improve sexual function if it is poor to start with. For more information on a healthy sex life and its links with CVD, see page 39.

What comes next?

Now you know the CVD warning signs and which apply to you the most, it's time to start making changes to your lifestyle to improve your health, longevity and enjoyment of life.

Read on for more in-depth information about the warning signs and vital statistics we've just discussed. When you're ready to start CLIP, go to page 59 for exercise advice and page 103 for the CLIP eating plan.

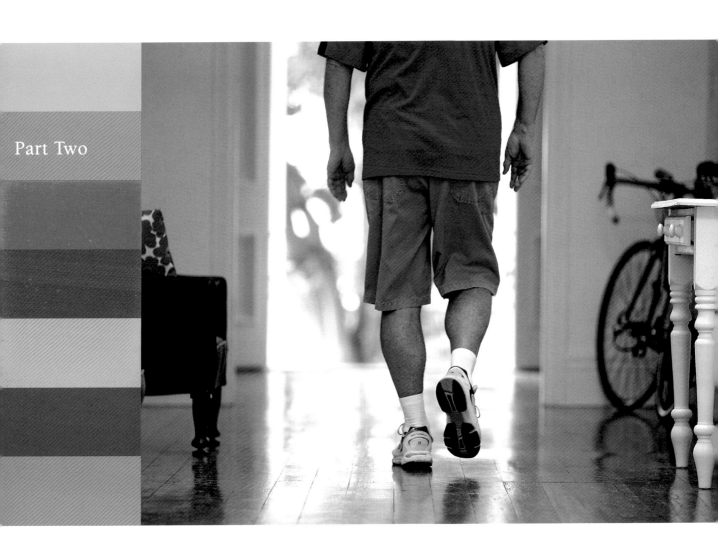

Part Two

Body, heart and mind

by Dr Manny Noakes, Dr Peter Clifton, Dr Grant Brinkworth,
Dr Jennifer Keogh, Adam Harrison, Dr Jane Bowen, Belinda Wyld,
Dr Phil Mohr and Dr Carlene Wilson

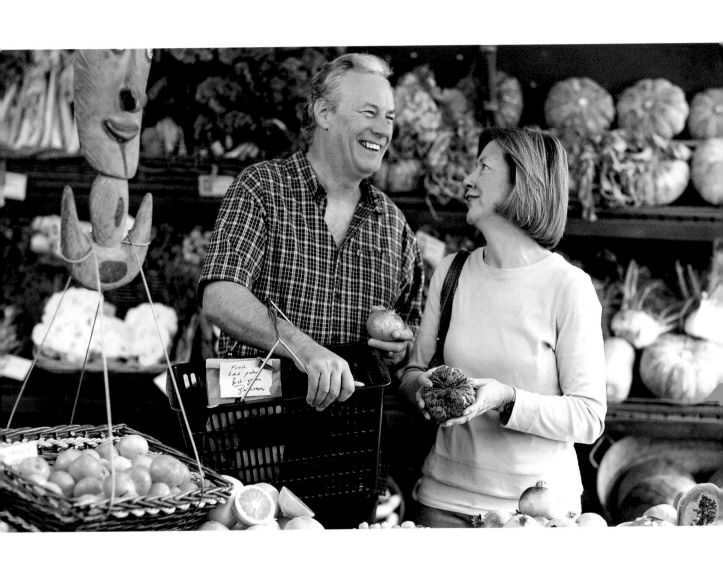

Weight and waistline

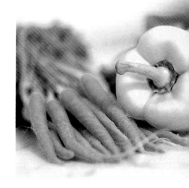

We all know that being overweight is bad for our health, but many of us still struggle to achieve and maintain a healthy body weight.

As we have seen, excess body fat increases the risk of CVD, high blood pressure, type 2 diabetes, osteoarthritis, stroke, sleep apnoea (see page 49) and many other conditions. These effects are greater when fat is stored mainly around the abdomen. Here are three reasons why being overweight can cause problems.

1   The bigger your body, the more work your heart has to do. A heart that requires more effort to pump blood also beats faster. This can increase your blood pressure.
2   The tubes to your lungs can be 'squashed' by the fat around your neck. This makes it more difficult to breathe while you sleep.
3   The fat in your abdomen becomes a source of excess fuel. The liver and blood are then flooded with fat and glucose they can't deal with. This causes fatty liver, diabetes and damage to the arteries that can result in stroke or heart attack.

Generally, younger men are more at risk of these complications than younger women, but as men age and women go through menopause, the risks become the same for both sexes.

The great news is that weight control can have many benefits. For some, better sleep patterns, better sexual health and improved self-esteem are just the beginning. Keep reading for an explanation of the fundamentals of body weight and weight loss, and some strategies for eating less.

How much weight should I lose?

The closer your weight is to the 'healthy' range, the healthier you will be, but you need to be realistic in setting your goals. Even losing 3–5 kilograms greatly reduces the risk of complications associated with being overweight *if it is maintained*. The aim is not to become 'thin', but to lose enough weight to improve your health.

Making permanent changes to your diet, engaging in regular activity and losing *some* weight will improve your health much more than a cycle of crash diets and returning to bad habits. See page 51 for tips on how to set yourself realistic goals. Once you have maintained a lower body weight for a few months you may want to plan another phase of weight loss.

How long will it take?

Generally, women (or men who are less overweight) should aim to lose 0.5 kilograms a week, while men (or women who are more overweight) should aim to lose 1 kilogram a week.

When you lose weight, three components of your body weight change: fat tissue, muscle tissue, and fluid or 'water'. To understand how quickly you will lose weight, it is useful to see how each of these changes as we lose weight.

Many people see the most dramatic decrease in weight during the first week or two of commencing a diet. This is because our bodies store a small amount of carbohydrate that has water attached to it, like a wet sponge. In the early stages of a diet, the body burns up this carbohydrate for energy, and the water attached to it is passed from the body. This water loss can produce a 1–4 kilogram reduction in body weight – and even more in some people. You should not, however, expect to continue losing weight at this rate.

After this early change, reducing your weight at an average rate of 0.5–1 kilogram per week (by combining a diet adequate in protein with exercise) encourages the loss of mainly fat and minimises the loss of muscle. This is important, not only because muscle burns more kilojoules than fat, but also because a higher muscle mass seems to be associated with living longer.

Differences in weight loss from week to week are perfectly normal, even if you follow the same eating and exercise plan. It is most useful to weigh yourself in the morning, after going to the toilet, wearing the same amount of clothing each time. Keep a record of your changing weight, BMI and waistline so that you can keep track of your progress.

How much less do I need to eat?

Reducing your food intake by about 2000 kilojoules a day should generally result in a weight loss of about 0.5 kilograms a week. Cutting your food intake by 4000 kilojoules a day should result in a weight loss of about 1 kilogram a week. To calculate what your kilojoule intake for weight loss needs to be, first calculate the number of kilojoules you need each day to keep your weight stable, then subtract 2000–4000 kilojoules. See 'Calculating your daily kilojoule requirement for weight loss' opposite for an example.

Once you have reached your target weight, you will want to maintain it. To do this, recalculate your kilojoule requirement based on your lower body weight and increase your food intake accordingly.

Some people, particularly older women who are less active and not very tall, may calculate that they need less than the basic 6000-kilojoule plan. If this is the case, we still suggest that you try the 6000-kilojoule plan, but bear in mind that you will lose weight more slowly. Alternatively, you could consult a professional dietician, who can adjust the plan to suit your needs.

The CLIP eating plan offers several different daily kilojoule totals, depending on what your daily intake should be. See page 109 for more information.

Calculating your daily kilojoule requirement for weight loss

Use the equations below to calculate your daily kilojoule needs. To do this you will need to select an activity factor from the table below, depending on how active you are.

activity level	description	activity factor
sedentary	desk job and little or no exercise	1.2
lightly active	light exercise or sport on 1–3 days a week	1.375
moderately active	moderate exercise or sport on 3–5 days a week	1.55
very active	hard exercise or sport 6–7 days a week	1.725
extremely active	hard daily exercise or sport or a physical job or hard training (for marathon, triathlon, etc.)	1.9

Women need to use the following equation:

$$[655.1 + (9.56 \times \text{weight in kilograms}) + (1.85 \times \text{height in centimetres}) - (4.68 \times \text{age in years})] \times 4.2 \times \text{activity factor}$$

Men need to use this equation:

$$[66.47 + (13.75 \times \text{weight in kilograms}) + (5 \times \text{height in centimetres}) - (6.76 \times \text{age in years})] \times 4.2 \times \text{activity factor}$$

example

Louisa is 57 years old, 158 centimetres tall, weighs 78 kilograms and does some light activity. Her BMI of 31.2 indicates that she is obese. Her daily kilojoule intake would be:

$$[655.1 + (9.56 \times 78) + (1.85 \times 158) - (4.68 \times 57)] \times 4.2 \times 1.375)$$
$$= [655.1 + 745.68 + 292.3 - 266.76] \times 4.2 \times 1.375$$
$$= 8240 \text{ kilojoules a day (rounded up)}$$

Louisa should aim to lose around 0.5 kilograms a week by cutting her kilojoule intake by 2000 kilojoules to about 6000 kilojoules a day. This is the kilojoule intake allowed on the basic level (level 1) of the CLIP eating plan (see page 108). Louisa should also aim to increase her activity by taking up regular exercise.

example

Martin is 50 years old, 180 centimetres tall, weighs 83 kilograms and has a sedentary lifestyle. Martin's BMI of 25.6 indicates that he is slightly overweight. To maintain this weight, his daily kilojoule intake would be:

$$[66.47 + (13.75 \times 83) + (5 \times 180) - (6.76 \times 50)] \times 4.2 \times 1.2$$
$$= [66.47 + 1141.25 + 900 - 338] \times 4.2 \times 1.2$$
$$= 8920 \text{ kilojoules (rounded up)}$$

If Martin wants to lose weight, he should aim to lose about 0.5 kilograms a week by cutting his food intake by 2000 kilojoules a day to about 7000 kilojoules a day. This daily intake is offered by level 2 of the CLIP eating plan (see page 109). He should also aim to take up a regular exercise program.

How can I make it easier?

There is no doubt about it – you will need to adjust to eating less food. There are a number of simple ways, however, to make this easier. CLIP includes each of the following strategies.

1   **Regular meals**

    If you know what you'll be eating and have planned your meals, this will help you to stay in control. Studies have shown that a regular meal rhythm is associated with long-term maintenance of weight loss. Unconscious nibbling, before or after meals, can provide a lot of excess kilojoules. Keeping a food diary can help you keep your eating in check.

2   **Protein-rich foods**

    These have been shown to reduce hunger. When we eat protein-rich food, hormones released from our gut tell our brain that we shouldn't feel hungry. It is important to include protein at all meals because this effect only lasts a few hours. Hunger is reduced after eating protein-rich foods such as lean red meat, chicken, fish, legumes or low-fat dairy foods.

3   **High-fibre foods**

    These include fruit, vegetables and wholegrain cereals. They increase your feeling of fullness and limit the amount of food you can eat in one sitting. For fibre to have this effect, you must eat slowly enough to allow time for the signal to travel from your full stomach to your brain. The old advice to chew your food thoroughly and eat slowly is worth following. Make sure you sit down at the table for all your meals. Some types of fibre can be particularly helpful in keeping your bowels regular. These are mostly insoluble fibre, such as that contained in wheat bran. Another type of fibre, soluble fibre, can help lower your cholesterol levels to a small degree (see page 95).

4   **Foods that contain water**

    These are more filling than foods from which the water has been removed. You will feel more full, for example, after eating three whole fresh apricots than you will after eating three dried apricots.

5   **Solid foods**

    These are more satisfying than liquid foods. Drink water if you are thirsty; eat solid food if you are hungry. Soft drinks, cordial, juices, beer and wine can be significant sources of kilojoules that do not satisfy hunger.

6   **Limited food options**

    Allowing yourself a large range of foods at each meal encourages overeating. Our volunteers say that eating similar foods at the same meal most days reduces the temptation to go for second helpings or extra-large servings. Eating similar breakfasts, morning teas and lunches on weekdays will take your focus away from food and eating. Variety is important when it comes to fruit and vegetables, but research shows that increasing the variety of meal options can encourage overeating.

7   **Smaller portion sizes**

    Almost all our volunteers say, 'I was taught as a child to finish everything on my plate and I still do, even if I'm full.' Many studies have shown that the amount we eat increases when the serving size gets bigger. Here are some very simple ways to break the habit of putting too much on your plate.

- Serve your meals on an entrée-sized plate.
- Cook only the required amount of food for the number of people you are feeding. If you are cooking for two but using the recipes in this book (which usually serve four), make the whole amount and freeze half for another meal. If you are cooking for one, eat a quarter and freeze the rest in three one-meal portions.
- When you are out and ordering food and drinks, avoid the temptation to order the larger size. Consciously choose the smallest size available or share a larger size with a friend.
- When eating in restaurants and cafés, order an entrée-sized meal.
- If you feel satisfied but haven't eaten everything on your plate, cover it and store in the fridge to eat another time.

Keep a checklist

During the early stages of a weight-loss program it can be very helpful to keep track of what you are eating. Many of the volunteers in our CLIP trials vouched for how useful this can be to help stay in control. See Appendix 3 (pages 261–62) for the CLIP eating plan daily checklist.

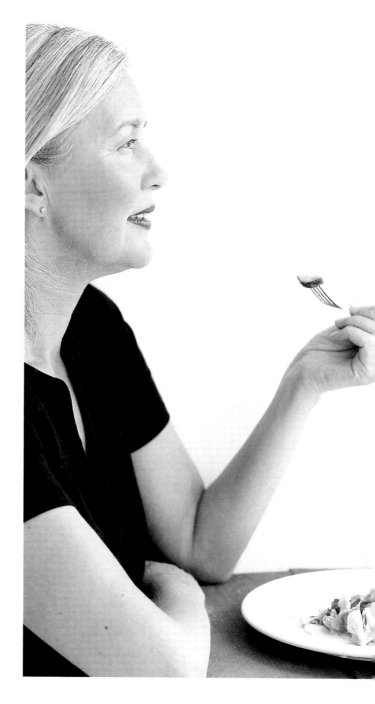

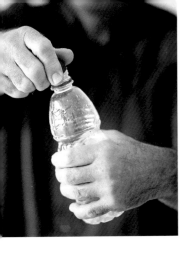

Cholesterol levels

Cholesterol is a waxy substance made in nearly all of our organs. High levels of the wrong kind of cholesterol are carried in our arteries and can lead to CVD and stroke.

Despite this, cholesterol is an essential part of the membranes surrounding our cells. Cholesterol is produced by all animals and carried around the body via the blood stream while contained within particles called lipoproteins. In small amounts, cholesterol is vital – it maintains cell membranes, and is used by our bodies to produce bile, some hormones and vitamin D. About three-quarters of the cholesterol in our bodies is made by us; the remaining quarter comes from food. Which foods we eat, in particular the type of fats that we eat, can influence how many cholesterol-carrying lipoproteins our body can produce.

There are two main types of lipoprotein that carry cholesterol. Whether cholesterol is considered 'good' or 'bad' depends on how the protein holds the cholesterol. 'Bad' cholesterol means low-density lipoproteins – LDL cholesterol – which are known to have a harmful effect on the arteries, while 'good' cholesterol means high-density lipoproteins – HDL cholesterol – which play a protective role.

If a blood test has shown that you have high levels of LDL cholesterol, you should bear in mind that your blood cholesterol is only *one* aspect of heart and blood-vessel health. Your cholesterol levels are important, but just how critical they are for your health depends on whether you also have other risk factors or already have heart disease or conditions such as type 2 diabetes. You can calculate your CVD risk by taking into account other risk factors, such as blood pressure and whether you smoke (see page 10). Whatever your situation, the lower your LDL cholesterol the better, especially if you have other risk factors.

Most blood tests for cholesterol will involve a 'lipid profile', which means the laboratory will measure your total cholesterol, LDL cholesterol, HDL cholesterol and triglycerides. Your total cholesterol reading is a rough measure of your CVD risk. The average total cholesterol level for Australians is around 5.4 mmol/L, but a healthier level is lower than this.

If your total cholesterol level is 6.5 mmol/L or more, your risk of CVD, including heart attacks and angina, is about *four times greater* than that of a person with a cholesterol level of 4 mmol/L.

Although many people with high cholesterol levels will not develop heart disease, if you discover your cholesterol level is high you must see your doctor and discuss plans to reduce your cholesterol levels and other CVD risks.

Your LDL cholesterol level is also an important marker; the lower the better. The Heart Foundation recommends an LDL cholesterol level of less than 2.0 mmol/L if you already have CVD.

Familial hypercholesterolaemia

The cause of your high cholesterol may be a genetic condition called familial hypercholesterolaemia (FH). If you do have FH, so may half of your brothers and sisters and half your children. About two in a thousand people have FH, but there are some ethnic groups, such as Afrikaners, Lebanese and French Canadians, among whom it is ten times more common than average.

FH causes early heart disease, especially in men; 50 per cent of men with FH will have had a heart attack before they are 50, so the sooner you find out whether you have it the better.

You are more likely to have FH if your total cholesterol is over 7.5. If you have cholesterol deposits in your Achilles tendons, on the back of your hands or below your knees, you definitely have FH. If you have high cholesterol and your close relatives also have cholesterol levels above 7.5, you should see your doctor to find out whether you have FH. Diagnosis may involve a genetic test.

If you are diagnosed with FH, your doctor will advise you to lower your cholesterol using both diet and medication. You should also make sure that your close relatives are tested as soon as possible.

Reducing your LDL cholesterol

There are two major causes of a high LDL cholesterol level: your genetic make-up, and your diet and lifestyle. Some drugs and certain medical conditions may also increase LDL cholesterol.

The foods that affect LDL cholesterol levels are those that are high in saturated fats. Saturated fats cause your liver to clear less LDL cholesterol from your blood, thus increasing your LDL cholesterol levels, which damages artery walls and promotes inflammation in the arteries. Diet can reduce your LDL cholesterol levels by as much as 20 per cent. The CLIP eating plan provides an appropriate diet for reducing your LDL cholesterol levels.

Saturated fats

Saturated fats are generally hard at room temperature. Examples are butter, copha, lard, full-fat dairy foods and the fat in meat. It's not just animal fats that are high in saturated fat. Palm oil, a vegetable fat that is often used in commercial baking, is also high in saturated fat, which is why a lot of the saturated fat in the Australian diet comes from cakes, biscuits, pies and pastries. Fatty foods such as sausages, fatty meats and chicken, and deep-fried foods cooked in beef fat, are also contributors. Until recently, many takeaway foods were cooked in highly saturated fat, but this is slowly changing.

How will you know what type of fat is being used? Ask the retailer what fat they use for cooking and how much saturated fat it contains. Less than 25 per cent saturated fat in cooking fats is reasonable.

Usually, fats that are liquid at room temperature are low in saturated fat and will contain healthy fats that

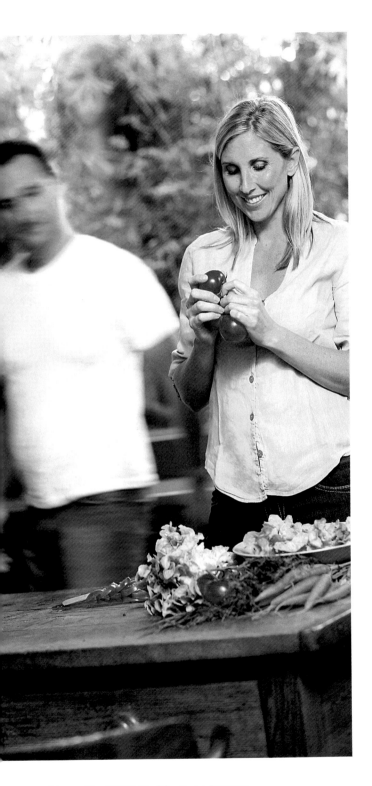

may help to lower your LDL cholesterol slightly. Foods containing these fats include olive oil, canola oil and soybean oil. The fats in nuts and avocados are also low in saturated fat.

Although these fats are certainly healthier for you, they have the same number of kilojoules or calories as saturated fats, so if you need to watch your waistline, don't be excessively liberal with healthy oils. On the other hand, certainly don't avoid healthy fats; they not only improve the taste of many foods including vegetables, they also provide many other protective nutrients.

If you are overweight and you lose weight, your total cholesterol level will generally go down and your HDL cholesterol will increase. You may find that, during active weight loss, HDL cholesterol will drop temporarily, but it will increase again after your weight has stabilised.

The CLIP eating plan provides a good amount of healthy fats and is low in saturated fat.

Trans fats

Not all unsaturated fats are good for you. Trans fats are partially hardened, unsaturated fats that not only increase LDL cholesterol but also lower HDL cholesterol and have been linked to heart disease. They are found in very low levels in beef and dairy fats as well as in some commercial baking and frying fats. Until the mid-1990s, trans fats were present in significant amounts in Australian margarines, but they have since been reduced to negligible levels.

If you choose lean and low-fat versions of beef and dairy foods, they will provide almost no trans fats and be low in saturated fat. Avoiding most commercial cakes, biscuits and pastries as well as commercially prepared deep-fried foods will generally guarantee that you will reduce your intake of both saturated and trans fats. The 'Tick' foods approved by the Heart Foundation contain the lowest possible levels of trans fats or none at all.

Foods enriched with plant sterols

A change of diet to reduce saturated-fat and trans-fat intake will lower LDL cholesterol by an average of about 10 per cent. If your LDL cholesterol levels are too high, however, a reduction of 10 per cent may not be enough. Plant-sterol-enriched foods – margarines and dairy products (see page 99) – could lower your cholesterol by another 10 per cent to a still healthier level.

Plant sterols are structural components of plants that resemble cholesterol in humans. They partially block the absorption of cholesterol by the body and thus lower LDL cholesterol. To enjoy the cholesterol-lowering effect of plant-sterol-enriched foods you must eat enough of them to ensure you ingest enough plant sterols. The CLIP eating plan will provide as many plant sterols as you need.

Cholesterol in eggs and prawns

Your LDL cholesterol levels are most affected by the amount of saturated fat you eat. Some foods also contain small amounts of cholesterol, which is absorbed in the small intestine and added to the cholesterol made by the liver. This dietary cholesterol increases blood cholesterol levels only slightly. Since foods that are high in cholesterol are usually also high in saturated fat, choosing low-saturated-fat foods such as low-fat dairy foods and lean meats will reduce your intake of dietary cholesterol.

Some low-saturated-fat foods, however, are particularly high in cholesterol – egg yolk, liver and shellfish, for example. But if you eat eggs as part of an overall healthy diet, research shows that up to 6 a week will not increase your CVD risk. Eggs are a rich source of many nutrients and an economical source of protein. Recent scientific results also show that 2 eggs can provide 132 mg long-chain omega-3 fatty acids (see page 93), which is a significant contribution to total daily intake of these important fats. Although prawns are also high in cholesterol, they are very low in fat and saturated fat. If you eat them on a regular basis, keep doing so, *but* make sure you steam or boil them, or cook them in an oil that is low in saturated fat rather than in a butter or cream sauce.

Increasing your HDL cholesterol

HDL cholesterol protects you from CVD by taking cholesterol away from the artery walls and helping to remove it from the body. Your HDL cholesterol can be increased by losing excess weight, drinking a moderate amount of alcohol and including more healthy fats in your diet. Exercise can also increase HDL cholesterol levels, but this is negligible for moderate exercise. Women tend to have higher HDL cholesterol levels than men.

Lowering your triglyceride levels

Triglycerides are another type of fat in the blood that indicate CVD risk. In addition to your genetic make-up, being overweight, overeating or having excess abdominal fat, poorly controlled type 2 diabetes or kidney disease can cause high triglyceride levels. A diet that is high in carbohydrates, especially refined carbohydrates such as those in white bread, rice, soft drinks, fruit juices and confectionery, can increase triglyceride levels as well.

Certain medicines can increase triglyceride levels. These include tamoxifen, steroids, beta blockers, some diuretics, oestrogen and contraceptive pills. Drinking a lot of alcohol can also produce high triglyceride levels.

To lower your triglycerides, reduce excess weight, increase your activity levels, drink alcohol only in moderation and reduce the amount of refined carbohydrate in your diet. The CLIP eating plan offers a combination of foods that will help you lower your triglyceride levels.

Medications for cholesterol control

Treatment of high cholesterol has been revolutionised in the last 20 years by the development of statin drugs, which can lower your LDL cholesterol levels by more than 50 per cent. They all partially stop the liver from making cholesterol, which draws cholesterol out of the blood and thereby reduces the risk of heart disease. The lowering of LDL cholesterol by 1.0 mmol/L reduces by 20 per cent the risk of heart disease or death from heart disease in the next 5 years. This great a change, however, is more likely if you have other cardiovascular risk factors.

Most people can take statins without experiencing any significant side effects, but some people, perhaps 10 per cent, develop muscle aches and pains that are sometimes so severe that they are forced to stop taking the drug. A tiny fraction of people suffer muscle 'meltdown', which can be very serious. This is more likely when the statin is combined with other drugs such as fibrates. Despite these rare side effects, however, statins have also been shown to reduce total deaths from heart disease, as well as the number of heart attacks.

Ezetimibe, which has appeared in the last few years, blocks the absorption of cholesterol from the gut and can lower total cholesterol by 20 per cent. The combination of a statin drug with ezetimibe is more effective than a statin alone and can lower LDL cholesterol by as much as 60 per cent. Ezetimibe has very few side effects and in combination with statins is very safe.

Fibrates are best at lowering blood triglyceride levels and elevating HDL cholesterol. They have not yet been proven to reduce heart disease significantly and they are not as strong as statins unless there is a triglyceride or HDL problem to start with. They can also help reduce fat in the liver, which may cause liver inflammation and cirrhosis.

The Pharmaceutical Benefits Scheme recommends the use of cholesterol-lowering medication by people who are at very high risk of CVD, no matter what their cholesterol level, in combination with a cholesterol-lowering diet. People who have high cholesterol but no CVD risk factors should follow a cholesterol-lowering diet for six weeks before having their cholesterol levels retested and their need for cholesterol-lowering medication reassessed.

Aspirin is often recommended for people who have suffered a heart attack or from unstable angina or stroke. Clinical trials show that aspirin helps prevent the recurrence of heart attack, hospitalisation for recurrent angina and second strokes. Aspirin also helps prevent such events in people who are at high risk. The risks and benefits of aspirin therapy vary for each person, so don't start without first consulting your doctor. If you are taking aspirin and you undergo a simple dental or surgical procedure, you must tell the surgeon or dentist your aspirin dosage.

Blood pressure

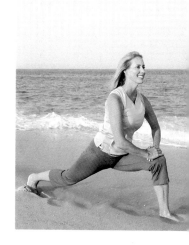

Blood pressure is the pressure caused by the blood circulating in the arteries as the heart pumps it around the body.

For all adults, the ideal blood pressure is less than $^{120}/_{80}$.

High blood pressure can cause serious problems, such as heart attack, stroke or kidney disease. It usually produces no symptoms so it is important to have your blood pressure checked regularly. If you need treatment for your blood pressure, the recommended target is usually less than $^{140}/_{90}$, but people with type 2 diabetes should aim for less than $^{130}/_{80}$.

Blood pressure tends to increase with age. If you have a family history of high blood pressure – that is, your mother, father, sister or brother had high blood pressure before the age of 60 – you are more likely to develop it too. It is a good idea to have your blood pressure checked at least once a year to make sure it is within normal levels.

Lowering your blood pressure

Lifestyle is important in helping to control high blood pressure. Losing weight, reducing your salt and alcohol intake and exercising regularly will all help keep your blood pressure within the normal range.

Losing weight reduces blood pressure by about 1 mmHg per kilogram of weight lost. This benefit may be only short-lived, however. Combining weight loss with a diet that is lower in salt prevents high blood pressure in the long term.

The link between salt intake and blood pressure is well known. Reducing salt intake can also reduce the need for blood pressure medication.

Watch your salt intake

Most people say they don't use much salt, which usually means they don't add salt to food. However, most processed foods contain salt, which makes it hard to avoid. About 75 per cent of our salt intake comes from foods such as bread, cereals and other processed foods. Australians eat about twice the amount of salt recommended by health authorities. The healthy salt target of

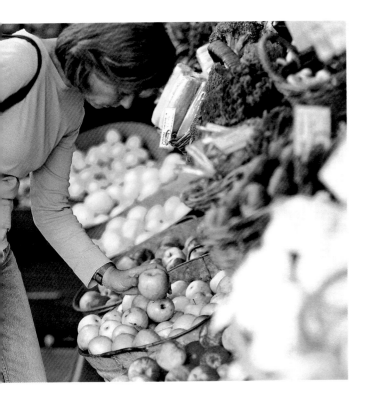

are just a few ingredients that will pep up your food without adding salt.

To lower the salt in your diet you can increase your intake of fresh fish, lean red and white meat, poultry, fresh vegetables and fruit, all of which are naturally low in salt. Frozen vegetables and fruit and tinned fruit are also low in salt. There are low- or reduced-salt alternatives available for tinned tomatoes, baked beans, sweet corn, tuna and salmon (in spring water or oil rather than brine, which is high in salt), and for packaged nuts.

When buying processed foods, try to choose foods with the Heart Foundation Tick; these are generally *lower* in salt (although not necessarily low-salt) than similar products without the Tick. Limit your intake of foods that are high in salt. These include:

- bacon, ham and some cheeses
- takeaway foods
- salted savoury snacks such as potato chips
- convenience foods such as instant soups, and
- condiments such as tomato, soy or chilli sauce.

And remember, sea salt, rock salt and vegetable salt are just as high in sodium as ordinary table salt.

Eat fruit and vegetables

Eating plans that include fruit, vegetables and low-fat dairy foods can help reduce blood pressure. Such diets may have a positive effect on blood pressure because they are higher in potassium as well as lower in salt. Potassium is found in many foods – fruit, vegetables, nuts, legumes and wholegrain cereals are all high in potassium. To keep up your potassium intake, try to include two serves of fruit and five serves of vegetables a day and choose wholegrain breads and cereals.

6 grams a day is achieved by only 6 per cent of Australian men and 36 per cent of Australian women.

Table salt is a chemical compound containing sodium and chloride. It is the sodium component that affects blood pressure, so the terms 'low-salt diet' and 'low-sodium diet' are often used interchangeably. The Australian Food Standards Code defines a low-salt food as one that contains less than 120 mg sodium per 100 g or 100 ml.

All manufactured foods must carry a Nutrition Information Panel showing the sodium content per 100 grams (mg/100 g) or 100 ml (mg/100 ml). To check if a food is low in salt, make sure that the sodium content is no more than 120 mg/100 g or 120 mg/100 ml.

Where possible we have reduced the amount of salt in the recipes provided in this book. Herbs, lemon or lime juice or zest, vinegar, garlic, pepper and chilli

The CLIP eating plan provides this number of fruit and vegetable serves each day, as well as adequate amounts of whole grains.

Choose lean protein foods

There is some evidence that a higher-protein diet that exchanges protein for carbohydrate helps lower blood pressure. High-protein foods include lean red meat, fish, chicken, pork, eggs, low-fat dairy foods, legumes and nuts. The CLIP eating plan offers a higher-protein option (Option 2), which we recommend if your blood pressure is high.

Choose fish rich in omega-3 oils

Fish and fish oils contain fats called omega-3 fatty acids that can reduce blood pressure. Fish oil supplements have been shown to reduce blood pressure but they need to be taken in very large amounts to have an effect. Reduced salt intake in combination with fish oil supplements has been shown to lower blood pressure more effectively than supplements alone. Including a daily fish meal in your weight-loss diet can also help reduce blood pressure more effectively than weight loss or fish intake alone. The CLIP eating plan includes fish twice a week at lunch and at dinner, controls salt intake and manages weight.

Low to moderate alcohol intake

There is an established link between alcohol and blood pressure. It is important to limit your alcohol intake to no more than 2 standard drinks (20 grams alcohol) each day for men, or 1 standard drink each day for women (10 grams alcohol). The CLIP eating plan allows moderate alcohol intake within these guidelines.

Regular exercise

Increasing physical activity can lower your blood pressure by as much as 10 mmHg. If your blood pressure is normal, exercise can prevent it rising as you age. If you are on blood-pressure medication, regular exercise could be enough to reduce your need for tablets.

For your exercise program to reduce your blood pressure, it must include aerobic activity. Examples are brisk walking, climbing stairs, jogging, cycling and swimming. Try and do at least 30 minutes of aerobic exercise on all or most days of the week.

The exercise program offered in this book includes both aerobic and strength-training exercise, and will help you increase fitness and lower blood pressure.

Some people swear by meditation as a means of lowering blood pressure and some studies agree, although it seems to depend on the form of meditation practised. A recent report suggests that the evidence is not strong enough to recommend general meditation as a treatment for high blood pressure. A specific form of meditation, however, known as transcendental meditation, has been shown to be very effective.

Medications for controlling blood pressure

If you are already taking blood-pressure-lowering medication, you are in a far better position than people were 20 years ago, when the drugs were limited and had nasty side effects. These days, most people do not experience any side effects.

In order to reduce your blood pressure to less than $^{140}/_{90}$ (or less than $^{130}/_{80}$ if you have type 2 diabetes) you may well need to take three different drugs. It is important to take your blood-pressure medication as advised by your doctor. Good blood-pressure control dramatically reduces the risk of stroke by 35–40 per cent as well as the risk of heart attack and heart failure. If you lose significant amounts of weight and change your lifestyle, your doctor may advise reducing your blood-pressure medication.

There are really four classes of blood-pressure-lowering medication, each of which has a different action and different side effects.

1 ACE inhibitors and angiotensin-receptor blockers

These are the most commonly used drugs for blood-pressure control today and have very few side effects. Sometimes the first dose, if too large, can cause a significant drop in blood pressure and thus dizziness. These drugs are very good for treating heart failure, and they protect the kidneys from damage in people with type 2 diabetes. In combination with a low-salt diet, these drugs are even more effective. Some people experience persistent coughing as a side effect of ACE inhibitors. If this occurs, your doctor may recommend that you take an angiotensin-receptor blocker (ARB) instead. Both ACE inhibitors and ARBs reduce blood flow in the kidneys, so these drugs must be used with care if you have impaired kidney function.

2 Diuretics or water tablets

These make you excrete more salt (and water), thus lowering your blood pressure by about 5 mmHg. Safe, effective and inexpensive, these medications have been used for many years and have been proven to save lives. Their only downside is that they tend to reduce the ability to deal with a sugar load, which can lead to type 2 diabetes or gout in some people. Both of these conditions are very rare among people who take the usual low dose.

3 Beta blockers

These have also been used for many years. They work by slowing your pulse rate and making your heart work less forcefully. They are also used to treat angina, heart failure and some disturbances in the heart's rhythm, and can save lives if used after a heart attack or heart failure. They should not be used if you have asthma. About 10 per cent of people have problems with tiredness and depression when taking beta blockers, and some men experience impotence.

4 Calcium-channel blockers

These are used to treat both high blood pressure and angina. They frequently cause swelling of the ankles at higher doses.

Blood glucose and type 2 diabetes

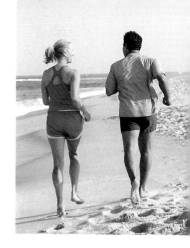

Type 2 diabetes is a condition in which the pancreas produces large amounts of insulin but the cells don't respond well to it, causing blood glucose levels to be much higher than normal.

Our bodies need energy for the various tasks we perform each day. They get this energy from a type of sugar called glucose. We break down complex carbohydrates from foods such as bread, cereals and fruit into glucose. As the glucose enters our bloodstream, the hormone insulin, which is made in the pancreas, helps to transport the glucose into our muscles and other cells, where it can be used for energy.

In some cases, the pancreas can no longer produce enough insulin, which results in high blood glucose levels. Too much glucose in the blood over a long period can cause hardening and narrowing of the arteries (atherosclerosis), which affects the blood supply to the heart and increases the risk of CVD. Prolonged high blood glucose levels can also cause serious damage to the kidneys, nerves and eyes.

Normally after we eat the carbohydrates in bread or pasta the glucose is released fairly rapidly and blood glucose levels rise, often peaking in 30–60 minutes. In response to carbohydrate in the gut and more glucose in the blood, insulin is released from the pancreas. This helps clear away the glucose so that after two hours glucose levels are returning to fasting levels.

If you have type 2 diabetes, you need a lot more insulin to clear the glucose, but because your pancreas cannot produce enough effective insulin to keep the glucose within the normal range, glucose levels remain high for a long time after a meal. In addition, your liver does not stop producing glucose after a meal, so glucose levels go even higher.

People with type 2 diabetes can stop eating all carbohydrates and still find their glucose levels are high because their liver makes glucose from other nutrients. Losing weight (or just eating less) dramatically reduces the glucose output from the liver.

Along with problems in controlling sugar levels, type 2 diabetes also causes an elevation of blood fats (triglycerides) and a reduction of HDL (good) cholesterol. If you have type 2 diabetes you need to keep an eye on both of these.

Diet

There are genetic causes for type 2 diabetes, so you're more likely to have it if your parents do. However, it is also very closely related to weight, so if you can stop or reverse weight gain, diabetes might never affect you even if both your parents have it.

To reduce your risk of eye and kidney disease, it is vital to lower your glucose levels. Controlling your blood pressure will also help prevent kidney disease. To prevent heart disease, you need to keep an eye on your glucose levels, blood cholesterol and triglycerides, and your blood pressure. Most people with type 2 diabetes die from heart disease, so you need to focus on prevention and/or management through weight control, diet and exercise.

Exercise

At all stages of diabetes, exercising will help. If you have diabetes, exercise dramatically improves your sugar and triglyceride levels. The exercise does not have to be strenuous; a bit of strength exercise can work wonders even if you are over 70.

Medication

Drug treatments fall into four main categories.

1   Insulin sensitisers

These drugs allow your body to use the insulin your pancreas can produce more efficiently. There are two major drug families in this category.

Metformin lowers blood glucose but cannot cause dangerously low glucose levels. It also results in minor weight loss. The major side effect is diarrhoea, and it cannot be used if your kidneys are starting to fail.

The glitazones (pioglitazone and rosiglitazone) can lower blood glucose dramatically while also lowering triglycerides, but they can cause quite large weight increases as well as fluid retention. They have not been shown to reduce deaths from heart disease, probably because they can lead to heart failure in some people. There may be differences between the two drugs in this respect, but the data are not yet clear. Both drugs are valuable in controlling blood glucose when this is urgently required to avoid kidney, eye or nerve damage.

2   Insulin releasers

These drugs cause the pancreas to produce more insulin in response to food and a rise in blood glucose. They can also lower blood glucose levels excessively, especially in very old people, for whom the doses may need to be lower, but this is relatively rare. Insulin releasers are available as long-acting drugs to be taken once a day or as tablets to be taken just before each meal. These tablets can cause weight gain.

3   Carbohydrate blockers

Only one of these is available, and it blocks the breakdown of carbohydrate in the gut, slowing the release of glucose and reducing the amount of glucose available for absorption. Instead, the carbohydrate travels to the large intestine, where bacteria break it down into gas and water. This leads to bloating and gas, which forces many people to stop taking the medication.

4   **Insulin**

At the moment, insulin can only be taken via injections (although inhaled insulin is on the way), so many people are reluctant to use it. It can, however, dramatically improve glucose and fat control, although this may require high doses. Often, very long-acting insulin is used as a basal treatment to control glucose production by the liver, with extra short-acting insulin to cope with post-meal rises. Many people manage on just the long-acting insulin in combination with other drugs. Although insulin may be a more natural treatment, it has not been shown to reduce deaths from heart disease. Insulin can cause weight gain, so for some people insulin releasers or insulin itself can lead to a vicious cycle of weight gain, increased insulin requirement and increased need for therapy.

People with lower long-term glucose levels (HbA1c) have a lower risk of heart attack. Of all the medications discussed above, only metformin has been shown to reduce deaths from heart disease.

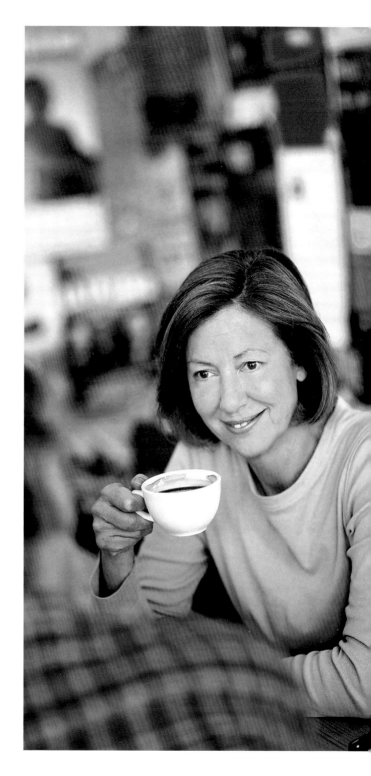

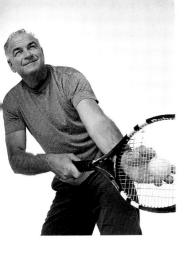

Exercise for a healthy heart

For a healthy heart, it is important to live a healthy lifestyle. This includes a balanced diet (such as the CLIP eating plan) and regular exercise.

Regular exercise is endorsed by the Australian Government and the Heart Foundation. In fact, regular exercise is one of the most important things you can do to improve your overall health and reduce your risk of CVD and other chronic diseases. Exercise can help improve a variety of health factors, including:

- reducing your body weight
- reducing abdominal fat
- improving your insulin sensitivity and glucose control
- reducing your blood pressure
- reducing your triglyceride and LDL cholesterol levels
- improving your fitness
- improving the health of your blood vessels, and
- significantly reducing your risk of early death, and of diseases that increase the risk of heart disease, such as type 2 diabetes.

Research has shown that exercise can reduce the risk of death from any cause and from stroke and heart attack. Regular exercise can substantially improve your health

no matter what your weight, even if you remain overweight (although losing a few kilograms will improve your health and reduce your risk of CVD even further).

Research has also shown that active people not only have fewer heart attacks but if they do have one, they recover faster and better than inactive people. Exercise also has many social and lifestyle benefits: active people are likely to feel more confident, happy, relaxed, have higher self-esteem, sleep better and experience an overall higher quality of life and level of satisfaction with their life.

Weights or walk?

Women often avoid muscle-strengthening exercise through fear that they will look masculine, or because they feel uncomfortable in the traditionally male-dominated weights room of the gym. Men often focus on strength work and forget about aerobic exercise.

Studies evaluating the effect of regular exercise on cardiovascular fitness have generally focused on aerobic exercise (such as brisk walking). They have shown that aerobic exercise is crucial in reducing the risk of heart disease and increasing longevity.

Research evaluating the impact of strength training on health is now building up, however. It shows that regular muscle-strengthening exercise is important for staying healthy and reducing the risk of heart disease. Strength training also allows people to maintain their independence for longer.

It is important to incorporate both aerobic and muscle-strengthening exercise into your exercise plan. The CLIP exercise plan offered in this book (see page 59) includes both forms of exercise in a simple and convenient program you can complete at home.

Australians and exercise

Participation rates in regular physical activity have declined in recent times and now over half of Australian adults (54 per cent, about 7 million Australians) do not regularly undertake sufficient physical activity to obtain a health benefit. In fact, over 2 million Australian adults (15 per cent) are termed 'sedentary', that is they do *no* physical activity at all. This leads to many health problems, which cost upwards of $370 million every year.

Daily activity and sedentary time

Becoming more active is important, whether it is by following a structured exercise routine or simply increasing your level of daily incidental activity.

We don't just need to do more exercise, we also need to live more active lives in general. Today, only a few jobs require vigorous physical activity, and most Australians engage in very little vigorous activity at work or during their leisure hours. The changes to our physical environment, labour-saving devices, such as cars, lifts, computers, household appliances and power tools, and greater access to sedentary leisure activities have all helped remove regular physical activity from our daily lives.

Sedentary occupations and sedentary activities, especially prolonged television-watching, independent of how much exercise we do, are directly associated with an increased risk of obesity and type 2 diabetes, both of which contribute to heart disease.

You will gain significant health benefits just by increasing your physical activity, such as cleaning, gardening, mowing, and so on. As long as you get slightly out of breath, the activity will be of benefit. Research has shown, however, that you can achieve even greater improvements in aerobic fitness, and extra protection against heart disease, as you add more exercise to your day and as your exercise becomes more vigorous. The more physical activity you do and the fitter you become, the lower will be your risk of CVD and premature death.

Exercise is for everyone

Daily, moderate-intensity exercise can lower your risk of CVD at any age. Most of us tend to become less active with age, and too often adults will sit and watch younger people be physically active when in reality we should all be participating.

In general, middle-aged and older people benefit from regular physical activity just as much as young people do. In fact, such activity increases the capacity of older people to perform daily activities and to maintain their independence. Almost immediately after beginning an exercise program, many older people notice that they feel better and find it easier to get around.

Recommendations for exercise

Health authorities recommend that we all do at least 30 minutes of moderate-intensity exercise on five or more days each week. Moderate-intensity exercise is anything that noticeably accelerates your heart rate, such as brisk walking. Regular moderate-intensity exercise can lower the risk of heart disease by 30–50 per cent. Participation in regular, vigorous physical activity

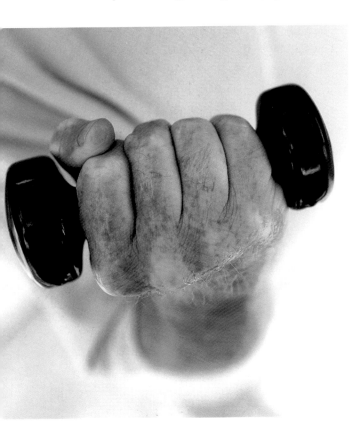

that makes you 'huff and puff', such as aerobics or jogging, will also improve your health and fitness and lower your risk of CVD even more.

If you are overweight and already physically active, it is important to stay active, even if you are not trying to lose weight. Physical activity is of great benefit to heart health, regardless of whether or not it is accompanied by weight loss. If you are inactive, the trick is to get started. People consistently cite a lack of time as their reason for not doing exercise. But it is possible to accumulate aerobic exercise in bouts of 10 minutes (that is, three or more 10-minute bouts) and achieve similar fitness improvements and health benefits to those you would gain from one continuous 30-minute exercise session. By splitting your exercise into short, separate sessions in this way, you'll find it much easier to fit exercise into your busy schedule.

You can probably find at least three 10-minute or two 15-minute pockets of time during your day. Find an activity you enjoy and then make it a part of your daily routine, just like eating, having a shower or cleaning your teeth. A few simple changes to your current schedule could give you this time. The activity checklist offered in this book (see page 258) is designed to allow you to plan multiple 10-minute blocks of activity each day. Opposite are some ideas for 10-minute activities you can do at home or work, in leisure time or while travelling. These make it easy to accumulate 30 minutes of moderate-intensity exercise each day.

As well as ensuring that you get enough physical activity, you should also aim to reduce the amount of time you spend on activities that do not require any large movements, such as sitting at the computer or watching TV. Such sedentary behaviours all contribute independently to the risk of CVD. Although they do not provide cardiovascular exercise, pushing a lawnmower, working in the garden or doing the vacuuming are all forms of exercise. If you do not have a job that requires physical activity, try taking the stairs rather than the lift, parking further away from your office or taking a brief walk at lunchtime. Even using fewer labour-saving devices, such as ride-on mowers, blenders or remotes, will help reduce your amount of sedentary time each day.

I'm too busy and tired for exercise

Many people think that exercise makes you tired. In fact, the opposite is true. Most people find that as they become more physically fit, their energy levels increase. Regular, moderate- to brisk-intensity exercise can also help reduce fatigue and manage stress. If you want to feel less tired all the time, three 10-minute blocks of moderate-intensity exercise a day could make all the difference.

Exercising at or near home

Here are some suggestions for making time in your day for exercise and/or for 10-minute physical activities that don't cost you anything or require you to go to a gym.

- Go for a bike ride as a fun way to improve fitness and explore your local area.
- Instead of spending 10 minutes finding a parking spot close to the shops, park your car at the far end of the car park and walk. Better yet, leave your car at home for short trips and walk or cycle there instead.
- Do household chores such as cleaning, vacuuming and dishwashing – they all count as physical activity.
- If you have a garden, get out there and prune, rake, weed and mow rather than pay someone else to do it.
- Reduce your sitting time. Watch less television and use the computer less. If you're watching television,

get up and jog on the spot for a 10-minute segment.
- Dance to your favourite upbeat music for 10 minutes a day.
- Create a new morning routine. Instead of spending time making and drinking your morning coffee, start your day with a 10-minute walk.
- Take your children or grandchildren outside to play and join in by kicking or catching a ball.

Exercising at work

Just because you're at work doesn't mean you can't get active. Here are some ways to fit in 10 minutes of exercise.

- Use the stairs rather than lifts or escalators.
- Replace your coffee break with a walking break.
- Take stretch breaks during meetings and when sitting in front of the computer. You could even have a 'walking' meeting: discuss work with a colleague while taking a walk.
- Get up and walk down the corridor to talk to a colleague instead of using the phone or email.
- Take a brisk walk at lunchtime for about 10 minutes.

Exercising during leisure time

- Join a tai chi, yoga or dancing class.
- Arrange to meet a couple of friends for a walk each day at the same time. If you all make a commitment to each other, you will be more likely to stick with it.
- Hit a tennis ball with friends or family.
- See how many different 10-minute activities you can find in your local area.
- If leisure for you means watching TV or a DVD, do it while you are exercising or stretching.

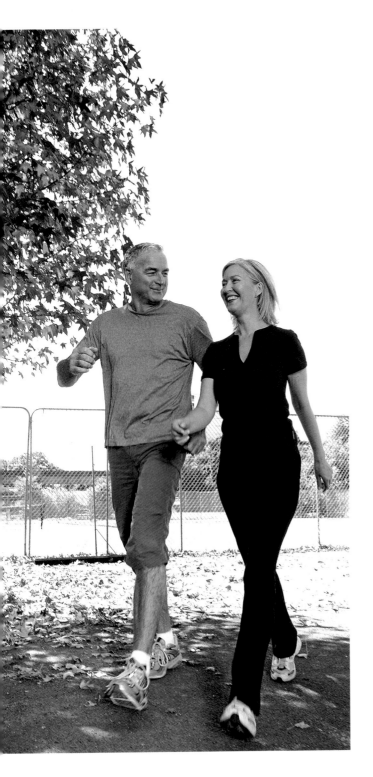

Exercising while travelling

- Walk or cycle to work. Apart from improving your health, you'll save money on petrol and help protect the environment.
- Get off the bus two stops early and walk the extra way to work or home. You will find it relaxing, particularly after a stressful day.
- Leave the car in a parking space 10 minutes away from work and walk the rest of the way.
- If your job involves a lot of driving, plan plenty of short stops during the day. Stop the car and walk for 10 minutes or more whenever you can.

Planning your exercise

The chart on page 258 offers a simple way to plan your 10-minute blocks of exercise. Many of the activities will just become habit after a while, such as getting off the bus early or parking the car a little further away. Plan your 10-minute 'snacks' of activity throughout the week; keep track of your activities and record your progress. For the full CLIP exercise plan, see page 59.

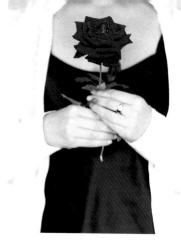

Sex matters

A good sex life is a predictor of good general health and wellbeing. Along with physical fitness and high levels of general activity, a good sex life has been shown to be important in happy ageing.

An American study showed that sexual activity in a loving relationship was associated with increased levels of social interaction and physical activity. All three of these factors helped protect people from age-related decline.

Carrying excess weight can affect us both physically and psychologically. One obvious mental health issue is body image, which in turn affects self-esteem. Depression, which can be related to body-image problems, can also damage your sex life and is certainly a risk factor for CVD. Excess weight can be linked to erectile dysfunction (ED) in men. High blood pressure, obesity, diabetes and heart disease can also have an impact on women's sex lives.

Improving your sex life

Here are some tips for maintaining a good sex life.
- Improve your fitness. This improves blood flow, general wellbeing and stamina.
- Maintain a healthy body weight.

- Control your blood glucose and cholesterol levels. High glucose levels contribute to tiredness and reduced desire. For men, nerve and blood vessel damage caused by long-term complications of type 2 diabetes and CVD can result in erection problems.
- Stop smoking. Smoking contributes to blood-vessel damage.
- Drink alcohol in moderation.
- Get adequate rest. It's hard to be in the mood when you're tired or stressed.

The treadmill or the bedroom?

There is an urban myth that sex is the best exercise you can do in terms of burning kilojoules. Unfortunately, while you can certainly work up a sweat, sex does not burn massive amounts of kilojoules. It is, however, a form of exercise, and even light-intensity exercise can improve your health.

Erectile dysfunction (ED)

Even in the age of Viagra, many men have difficulty talking about ED, and some younger men are even too embarrassed to seek help. Yet research shows that ED is surprisingly common. Rates of ED vary from 1–9 per cent for the under-40s, to as high as 20–30 per cent for men aged 40–59, 20–40 per cent for men aged 60–69, and 50–75 per cent for men in their 70s and 80s.

Problems with blood flow, nerves, hormone imbalances and psychological factors can all lead to ED. The heavier and less fit you are, the less responsive your blood vessels become. Narrowing of blood vessels, referred to as atherosclerosis, can affect blood flow, and adequate blood flow is vital for developing and maintaining a good erection. The problems with blood flow that can cause ED are the same ones that can cause heart disease.

While the severity of erection problems may vary, ED is usually associated with poorer emotional and relationship health. There seems to be a domino effect: as our sex life suffers, so does our self-esteem and quality of life. Men who attempt sex unsuccessfully are less likely to try again. Comments from a European survey of approximately 3000 men who currently have or previously have had ED highlight that erection problems can be a source of stress for many men.

- Overall, almost 55 per cent of the men in the study agreed that 'the erection problem is a source of great sadness for me'.
- About 53 per cent felt that this was also a source of great sadness for their partners.
- Almost 44 per cent agreed that 'hardly a day goes by that I do not think about this problem'.
- Only 50 per cent agreed that they and their partner were able to 'work around the erection problem'.
- Only 42 per cent were aware of 'other ways to get sexual gratification that did not require a good erection'.

ED and heart disease

It is becoming clearer that ED can be an early warning sign of heart problems. Recent research on the links between ED and heart disease showed that in 67 per cent of study volunteers, erection problems began an average of three years before they were diagnosed with heart disease. It is estimated that 50–70 per cent of men with CVD have also experienced ED. The link between ED and CVD is becoming so compelling that there may be a case for patients with erection problems being automatically checked for their vascular health as well. A decline in health can also lead to depression, which is strongly related to sexual problems. Studies show that 20–30 per cent of patients with heart failure have also been diagnosed with depression.

It is common knowledge that being overweight can lead to diabetes, which is also a strong predictor of sexual and erection problems. Indeed, ED can occur ten to fifteen years before a man is diagnosed with diabetes. Some drugs prescribed for high blood pressure may make it more difficult to have and sustain an erection. The drugs used to treat erection problems, however, such as sudenafil (Viagra), can be dangerous in combination with some heart medications, such as the nitrates used to treat angina. It is important to speak with your doctor if you are experiencing ED, to ensure that your medication strikes a balance between looking after your heart and your sex life.

What you can do

Whether you are a man or a woman, you should discuss any problems with sexual arousal with your doctor, to establish possible causes and suitable treatment. If you are overweight or obese, losing weight and engaging in regular exercise can generally partially restore sexual function. An American study showed that men who don't exercise could reduce their risk of ED by walking briskly for a little over 3 kilometres a day.

Diet can also help. A study examining the efficacy of a Mediterranean dietary pattern showed that men who followed this diet enjoyed significant improvements in cholesterol, glucose and insulin levels, as well as blood pressure. As a consequence, approximately one-third of the men on the diet regained completely normal sexual function. These changes were related to increased intake of fruit, vegetables, nuts and legumes, and to an improved ratio of polyunsaturated to saturated fats in the diet. The CLIP eating plan offers a similar balance of healthy foods.

A CSIRO diet-based intervention study showed that weight loss was associated with increases in both sexual desire and erectile function. The positive mental health effects of restoring erectile function can also be substantial.

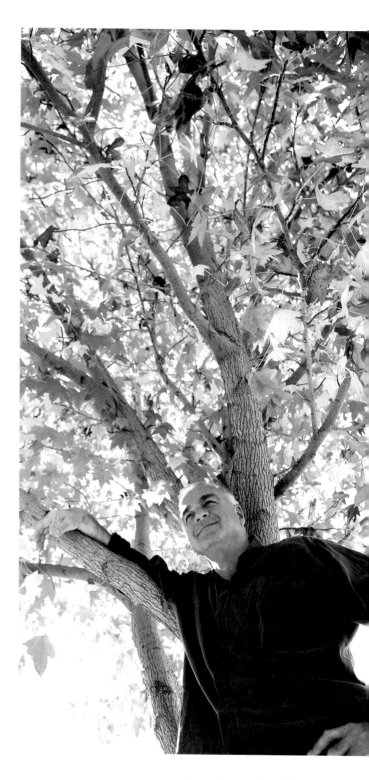

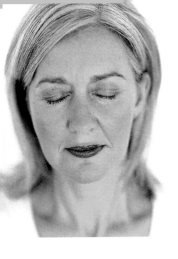

Depression and dealing with stress

The experience of stress is normal and common. In fact, we need a certain amount of stress to help us push our boundaries, avoid boredom and achieve peak performance.

The idea that stress can cause CVD is controversial, but since perceived stress can affect our quality of life, it is important to learn how to manage stress.

Usually when we talk about stress, we are referring to a gap between our problems and our abilities to cope with them. The greater this imbalance, the greater our experience of stress. While some stress (known as eustress) can be beneficial, any stress that is related to depression, social isolation or a lack of quality social support can be a significant risk for our health.

Our bodies have a natural instinct to recognise and respond to stress – it is what keeps us alert and prepared for danger. But the actual physiology of stress is a complex interaction between our nervous system and the production of hormones.

When we perceive stress, our nervous system activates various parts of our body to produce a range of chemicals, such as adrenalin, the 'fight or flight' chemical. Adrenalin helps boost the supply of blood to the brain, heart and muscles and releases glucose to give us an energy boost. Our body also prepares to resist the impact of stress. For example, the hormone cortisol increases blood sugar and blood pressure and suppresses our immune system to help reduce inflammation.

The effect of the chemicals released by the nervous system is usually rapid and lasts only for a short time. However, the hormones produced in response to stress react more slowly and their action persists for longer. It is the interplay between these two systems in our bodies that forms the basis of our stress response, as well as creating the potential for stress to lead to illness.

Understanding how our bodies react to stress does not completely explain what stress is, however. This is because it is both a psychological and a physiological response.

The causes of stress

Stress can be caused by anything that forces us to adjust to our changing environment. This could be something linked to outside factors, such as government policies, a change in the environment in which we live or work, or our personal relationships. Stress can also stem from our lifestyle choices, attitudes and feelings, or unrealistic expectations. Exactly what causes stress is different for everyone, as we all have our own unique set of coping abilities and can react very differently to the same events or demands, which are known as stressors.

The types of stressors we are most familiar with are frustrations, conflicts and pressures. Frustrations are those unpredictable events that get in the way of us achieving our goals or meeting our needs: when we're caught in peak-hour traffic on our way to work, we misplace our house keys, or we can't sleep because our neighbour is having a party. Frustration stressors can also arise when we feel we lack the abilities we need to fulfil a task or when we tell ourselves that we simply aren't good enough, smart enough or young enough. This type of self put-down is known as negative self-talk.

Conflicts arise when we find ourselves in situations in which we must make a decision based on options that seem incompatible. The options could be desirable (such as choosing between two job offers that both present you with career advancement), or unfavourable (for example, choosing between quitting your job and being laid off), but they both cause stress.

Pressures, on the other hand, are based on what we think others expect from us as well as demands we place on ourselves. We experience pressures, for example, when we feel compelled to work long hours in order to please our boss, feel we must maintain a clean house and tidy garden, or feel forced to be a loyal team member, a perfect parent or a self-funded retiree.

Factors such as our personality, coping skills and social network can all affect what we consider to be a stressful event. Our emotional and physical well-being can be unbalanced not only by the actual source of the stress, but by our perceived lack of resources to cope with the stress. Stressors that originate from an important part of our life (such as our relationships or occupation), or that continue to be a problem over time, will cause the greatest disruption. The more life changes or personal challenges we face at once, the more intense the stressful experience will be.

Types of stress

Stress can be divided into two main categories: acute and chronic.

1 **Acute stress**
   Acute life-event stressors can trigger CVD events. Acute stressors include significant life events, such as a bereavement, and catastrophic events, such as an earthquake or a terrorist attack.

2 **Chronic stress**
   Chronic stress produces long-term and negative reactions to the demands and pressures of our lives, but its effects on CVD vary. It can stem from such things as financial worries, strained relationships, bullying or harassment, fearful living situations or the strain of caring for an elderly parent. Chronic stress that is related to social disadvantage, social isolation or lack of social support is strongly associated with CVD.

Symptoms of stress

Stress affects our body, our mind and our behaviour in many ways. Just as the reaction to stress varies from one person to another, so too will the degree to which stress symptoms affect our health, emotional wellbeing and relationships. If you notice more than one of the changes in the table on page 46, you should see your doctor.

When stress becomes a problem

The 'fight or flight' reaction that our body initiates in response to stress is designed to keep us safe in the face of danger and to enhance our abilities to escape that danger. Although the stressors in our modern world pose more of a psychological than a physical threat, our body can't tell the difference. Whether we are threatened by violence or speaking in public, our body will release the same chemicals to heighten our awareness, sharpen our skills and enable us to survive.

Stress becomes a problem when our body's response is continually stimulated. The more the stress response is activated, the harder it is for the body to return to a resting state and revive itself. It takes energy and resources to initiate and maintain a stress reaction. It is no surprise then that the longer the stress hormones and increased sugar circulate in your blood, and the longer your heart and blood pressure remain elevated, the more damage is done.

The effect that chronic stress has on our physical health and emotional wellbeing has been well documented, and some studies suggest that over two-thirds of all illnesses could be stress-related. Recent research suggests that long-term stress can trigger or aggravate the following health problems:

- hypertension and heart attack
- cancer
- diabetes
- depression
- eating disorders
- obesity
- irritable bowel syndrome
- substance abuse
- memory loss, and
- infertility.

Our unique reactions to stressful events, together with our personality and even gender, mean it's difficult to determine exactly how our health will be affected by stress. One person may react with memory loss and depression, while another may develop irritable bowel syndrome.

Despite these differences in how people respond to longer-term stress, it is important to learn to recognise and manage those situations that trigger your stress responses before it becomes a real problem.

Managing stress

The key to coping with all types of stress is to understand which stressors are the most problematic, and learn ways to deal with them effectively. As some stress is beneficial to our wellbeing, the goal of stress management is not to eliminate stress but rather to learn strategies that will help us use it to optimise our performance. The great thing about dealing with stress is that we can teach ourselves how to do it.

The first step in managing your stress is to note how you react when you feel stressed. Does your chest feel tight? Do you hold tension in your neck and shoulders? Do you dread getting out of bed? Do you cancel outings with friends or snap at everyone around you? It is important to listen to these early signs, because if you ignore them, your mental, emotional and physical health could suffer.

Just as our stress responses are personal, so too are our coping strategies. What is relaxing for one person may be boring or stressful for another. Once you understand how you react in a stressful situation, you can begin to identify ways to cope with that stress that feel right for you.

Although people deal with stress in many different ways, when learning to manage your own stress it can be difficult to know where to start. You might like to try some of the ideas below next time you feel stressed.

1 Breathe!

Sometimes when we get stressed our bodies become physically tense and our breathing becomes shallower. Next time you feel your body stiffen in response to stress, take a minute or two to concentrate on your breathing. Breathe deeply in through the nose and out through the mouth, counting to ten with each breath in and out.

2 Learn positive self-talk

It's easy to become pessimistic when we're stressed, and often we fall into the trap of criticising our decisions, telling ourselves we aren't good enough or that we deserved what happened, and tarnishing every aspect of life with our negative responses. Positive self-talk is one of the most beneficial skills we can learn to manage our stress.

When you next experience stress, notice how your mind responds to the situation and write down any negative thoughts or feelings that come into your head. Then try to turn each point into a positive and say it aloud, silently or write it out again until you notice a shift in how your mind and body are responding.

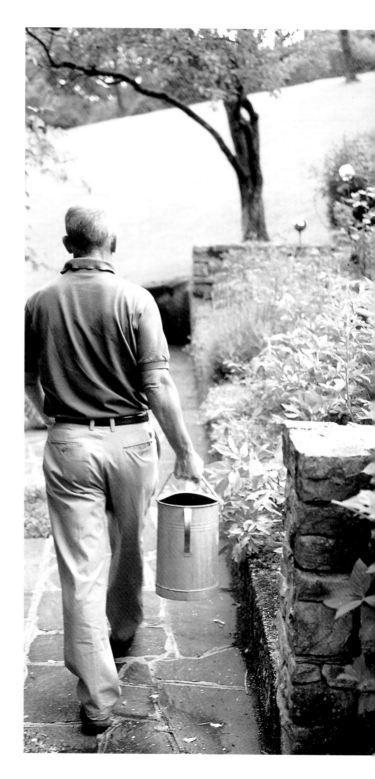

3 **Recognise what you can change**

An important part of managing stress is to put it into perspective and recognise what you can and can't change and what is worth fighting for. Don't waste time worrying about things that are out of your control, or planning for the worst.

4 **Do something relaxing**

Stress brings tension and pressure into our lives, and a good way to keep these symptoms in check is to slow down when you can and make time for activities you enjoy.

Go for a walk along the beach, take the kids for a walk through the park, go swimming, curl up on the couch with a good book, soak in a bubble bath or get a massage. You may like to put on your favourite CD, watch the world go by over a cup of coffee, or simply do nothing. Some people use relaxation techniques, meditation or tai chi to calm their mind and body and bring a sense of peace and balance to their life. Transcendental meditation is a specific form of meditation that has been shown to reduce blood pressure effectively. Having a hobby is also a great way to keep stress in check, and can connect you with people who have similar interests.

Whatever activity you choose as your 'time-out' from the pressures and demands of your working and personal life, make sure it provides you with the rest and relaxation you need to recharge your batteries.

5 **Laugh!**

Sometimes laughter really is the best medicine. Maintaining a sense of humour and the ability to laugh at yourself can lift your spirits, alleviate tension and keep you feeling relaxed and happy.

6 **Exercise regularly and maintain a balanced lifestyle**

One of the best ways to deal with stress is to enjoy regular physical activity. This is because exercise releases chemicals (called endorphins) that make us feel better, happier and naturally energised. This doesn't necessarily mean taking a structured fitness class at the gym – why not take the dog for a walk, spend some time in the garden, wash the car or play with your children or grandchildren?

Signs and symptoms of stress

physical symptoms	thoughts	behaviours	feelings
headache	memory problems	irrationality	general moodiness
back/neck pain	lack of concentration	withdrawal	anger
heartburn/reflux	indecisiveness	nervous habits (e.g. biting nails)	irritability
diarrhoea	confusion		anxiety
irritable bowel syndrome	lack of thought clarity	excessive exercise	depression
rapid heartbeat	racing thoughts	alcohol and drug abuse	apathy
sweaty palms	negative self-talk	changes in eating and/or sleeping patterns	loss of enthusiasm
high blood pressure	escapism	short temper	teariness
shortness of breath	decreased self-esteem		clumsiness
weight gain or loss	self-criticism		
cold or flu	forgetfulness		
fatigue			

It is also important to take care of yourself by eating well and getting adequate sleep. When we are stressed it is easy to give in to our cravings for chocolate, chips or ice-cream. Unfortunately, these comfort foods can do more harm than good, feeding our bodies with more sugar and fat than we need and making us feel sluggish. Well-nourished bodies are better equipped to cope with stress.

7 Be organised

When we are stressed, we can become forgetful, feel like our thoughts are scattered and find it difficult to concentrate. An easy way to manage stress is to keep a diary or 'to do' list with all your deadlines, appointments, tasks and commitments. To make sure you have time to unwind and relax, be sure to schedule in some 'you' time. Give priority to the most important activities and gradually work through your list. Keep in mind that you should review your list regularly. This will help you keep your life organised and ensure you manage your time in the best possible way.

8 Talk it out

Talking about our feelings and thoughts with people we trust can help us see our problems in a different light. By giving us clarity of thought and the opportunity to imagine different solutions, talking about stress can actually improve our reaction to it and help us to focus on solving our problem. 'A problem shared is a problem halved' is a good saying to remember.

9 Learn to say no

We are all guilty of taking on more responsibilities and commitments than we can handle. When we do this, we cause ourselves more stress, because we make our lives even busier and more chaotic. Stop trying to please everyone and learn to say no without feeling guilty about your limits.

10 Know when you need help – and get it

Sometimes stress can become such a consuming experience that we simply have no idea how to cope and keep a healthy balance in our life. Recognise when stress becomes a problem for you and don't be afraid to seek professional help. You may even be depressed and not know it. Visit www.beyondblue. org.au and check your depression score.

Stress and CVD

When we look at the physiology of the stress response, we can see why researchers have long thought that stress may affect the heart. During stressful situations, our heart requires more oxygen because of the increase in our heart rate, which can lead to angina, and our blood pressure rises due to the release of adrenalin, which can injure our artery walls. The number of blood-clotting factors circulating in our blood also increases in preparation for injury, and this can raise the risk of blood clots forming. It has commonly been thought that atherosclerosis, hypertension, stroke and heart attack can be attributed to these responses.

Understanding the link between stress and CVD, however, is not that simple. It is complicated by the fact that people mean different things by the term 'stress' and that the perception of and response to stressful events varies from person to person.

While our knowledge of the relationship between stress and CVD is still emerging, research has shown that some forms of stress *do* play a role in many heart-related disorders. An expert working group of the Heart Foundation concluded that there is compelling evidence for a causal link between certain foundations of stress, such as depression, social isolation and lack of quality social support, and CVD. The same report also concluded, however, that there is no consistent evidence for a causal link between chronic life events, work-related stressors, type A behaviour patterns, hostility, anxiety disorders or panic disorders, and CVD.

Research has consistently shown that our chance of developing CVD is increased if we smoke, have high blood cholesterol, do not exercise, have diabetes or high blood pressure, are overweight, depressed, socially isolated or lack social support. As many of the risk factors for heart disease are also signs or symptoms of stress, it becomes difficult to disentangle the relationship and prove that stress *causes* coronary events. What makes matters more complex is that personal factors (such as lifestyle, coping style, mood and personality) can either decrease or contribute to the risk of CVD.

While managing stress makes sense for our overall health, stress reduction as a therapy for CVD has not been scientifically proven. Most of us would agree, however, that managing stress can improve our quality of life. Maintaining regular physical activity and a balanced diet are particularly important stress-management tools because they are cardioprotective; that is, they're good for your heart.

Like most stress-related health conditions, CVD is largely preventable. By learning to manage our response to stress effectively, we may not only be improving the health and wellbeing of our minds and bodies, but we may also be helping our hearts.

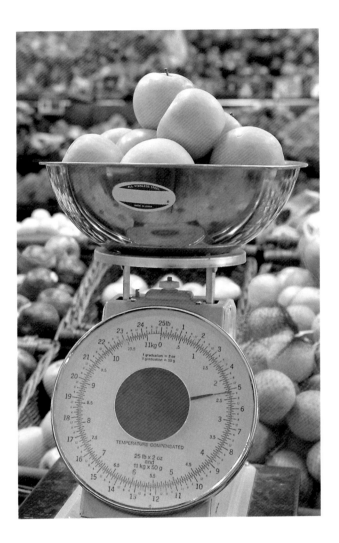

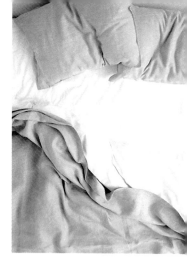

Sleep apnoea and a good night's sleep

We all feel much better after a good night's sleep, but recent research shows just how important sleep can be for our health, in particular our heart and circulation.

Anyone who has had an interrupted night's sleep knows only too well its effects on mood, concentration and general wellbeing the next day. Sleep is a period of rest and repair for the body as well as the brain. Lack of sleep is associated with higher blood pressure, since when we sleep our heart slows down and our blood pressure drops for several hours.

Research has shown that, compared with people who sleep 7–8 hours a night, people who sleep less than 5 hours a night also exercise less and are more likely to carry excess weight and to suffer from type 2 diabetes and depression. Lack of adequate sleep has been shown to increase appetite and levels of blood glucose and insulin, which can contribute to developing excess weight.

These issues can become a vicious circle, as being overweight can also lead to a sleep disorder called sleep apnoea (see page 12). Lack of sleep can in turn lead to lethargy and lowered energy levels, which can reduce physical activity. Sleep apnoea is more prevalent in men and increases with age. If you think you may have sleep apnoea, you should seek immediate medical attention.

The risks of untreated sleep apnoea include heart attack, stroke, impotence, irregular heartbeat, high blood pressure and CVD. You may have sleep apnoea if you suffer:

1 headaches when you wake up
2 tiredness, despite having slept
3 hypertension, and
4 a tendency to fall asleep when you should be awake.

If you snore, ask other people about your snoring patterns. You may have sleep apnoea if your snoring builds up to a peak, followed by a period of not breathing, after which your snoring starts again in a cycle that is repeated every 30–60 seconds.

A sleep test is usually required to diagnose sleep apnoea. Treatment is vitally important, because lack of sleep can cause daytime drowsiness and increase the risk of motor-vehicle accidents. In many cases, weight loss alleviates the symptoms. Moderate-to-severe sleep apnoea is usually treated with a C-PAP (continuous positive airway pressure), a machine that blows air into the nose via a nose mask while you sleep. This keeps the airways open and unobstructed. In some cases, surgery can relieve symptoms.

When we sleep and how much sleep we need are determined by our exposure to light. Exposure to daylight turns off our sleep hormones. When the sun sets, our sleep hormones are released and build up until we are tired enough to sleep again; this is called the circadian rhythm. Unfortunately, our modern lifestyle gives us many opportunities to override our body clock and extend the amount of time we are awake. This means that many of us are either not getting enough sleep or that the sleep we do get is not of good quality.

Several nights of insufficient sleep can affect the hormones that control appetite, causing us to crave high-fat, sweet foods. Researchers have found that people who sleep less than 6 hours or more than 10 hours a night are more likely to be overweight and to have high cholesterol and increased blood pressure, all of which are risk factors for CVD. The optimum amount of sleep for most adults is between 7 and 9 hours, so we all need to rethink our late nights.

Answer the following questions to see whether you need to change your approach to sleep.

1 Do you have an irregular bedtime or get up at a different time each day?
2 Does it regularly take you longer than 15 minutes to drop off to sleep?
3 Do you find it hard to get back to sleep after waking up during the night?
4 Do you take sleeping tablets to help you sleep?
5 Do you ever drink alcohol to help you sleep?
6 Do you regularly watch TV or talk on the telephone while you're in bed?

If you answered yes to any of these, you may like to try the following tips for getting a better night's sleep.
• Listen to your body clock and work with it.
  * Get up at the same time every day – a regular routine will help reset your internal clock.
  * Don't ignore tiredness – go to bed.
  * Don't force sleep – if you're not tired don't go to bed until you are.
  * Sleep in at weekends if possible – experts now acknowledge that it is possible to 'catch up' on sleep.
  * Get out in the sunshine – this is especially important in winter.
• Make sure your sleeping environment promotes good sleep.
  * Have a comfortable bed.
  * Make sure your bedroom is not too hot or cold.
  * Block out noise – buy earplugs if you have to.
  * Associate your bedroom with rest and relaxation – remove the clutter and the TV.
• Avoid drugs, alcohol and cigarettes.
  * Sleeping pills should only be taken as a temporary measure under medical supervision.
  * Alcohol disturbs the natural sleep rhythm, reducing the quality of your sleep.
  * Cigarettes stimulate the nervous system, increasing your heart rate and blood pressure, and keeping you awake.

Note that if these tips don't help, you may have a serious sleep disorder that requires the help of a specialist.

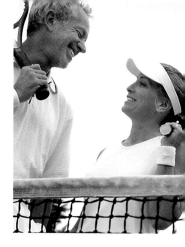

Motivation – mind over matter

Taking control of your health demands commitment to a lifestyle that will both decrease your risk of CVD and improve your wellbeing. Here are some strategies that should help you achieve this lifestyle change.

1 Set yourself realistic goals

The first step on the path to a healthy lifestyle is to develop realistic goals. You may wish to set your expectations in consultation with your doctor, but they will help you most if you set them yourself. You should set goals that are realistic and achievable, but also challenging and motivating. Your goals should neither be so small as to be meaningless nor so big as to set you up for failure.

Once you have set yourself a specific weight-loss or exercise goal, you should establish a plan for achieving it. But once you have done so, you need to have more goals in place for maintaining your weight, cholesterol levels or exercise routine.

Another important step is to make your goals concrete: write them down. You should include a description of the what, where and when of your eating plan and lifestyle changes. Then place the plan in a prominent position to remind yourself of what you want to achieve. You should also aim to reward yourself once your goal has been attained. See point 4 for more on the importance of monitoring your performance and rewarding yourself whenever you reach one of your goals.

Goal-setting is even more helpful if you think about the timeline for achieving your goals, and consider circumstances and events that might hinder or help your efforts. For example, don't plan to cut your food and alcohol consumption in the week before Christmas or to join a gym just before an overseas holiday.

Research suggests that men have more difficulty than women in being realistic about weight-loss and exercise goals. But whoever you are, discussing your goals with someone close to you will help. It will allow you to develop a plan that fits your needs and those of your family and friends. And a lifestyle that can be shared by the family is more likely to succeed.

2 Be active in a fun way

Losing weight initially depends a great deal on your ability to moderate your energy intake, but your chances of sustaining your success will be greatly enhanced by a commitment to regular exercise. This doesn't mean you have to join a gym or a sports group, although these are good strategies. What is important is to commit to being more active on an ongoing basis, which will require you to find an activity you enjoy doing and make it a high priority. You should devise concrete plans for how you will incorporate the activity into your life.

One solution is to make exercise something you do as a matter of routine, rather than something you have to go out of your way to do. You could consider getting rid of the second car and using a bicycle as back-up transport, for example, or committing to regular exercise with a friend or colleague, such as a walk at lunchtime. You don't have to be a sports star, just decrease the time you spend not being active.

The best thing about exercise is that it becomes more fun and easier to do as time goes on. Exercise generally has a positive effect on how you feel, so that many challenges in other areas of your life seem easier to face. Your initial challenge will be to view your time commitment to exercise as an investment in your future rather than a cost in your present.

3 Maintain regular mealtimes

It is very tempting to try to lose weight quickly by skipping meals. Many people routinely skip breakfast, for example, substituting morning tea or lunch. Although weight loss does require reducing your kilojoule intake, you can manage this easily without forgoing any meals. Successful strategies for doing this include reducing your portion sizes, the frequency of your snacks and the kilojoule content of your snacks and meals.

Your strategies should not be so extreme, however, that it is impossible to adhere to them. There is no value in committing to restraint that verges on starvation and is not only impossible to sustain long-term but also dangerous. Research shows that people who are successful at maintaining weight loss are those who reduce, rather than eliminate, their intake of high-fat and high-sugar foods, including fast food. These people are described as having 'flexible control' of their eating behaviour and studies indicate that flexible control is critical to maintaining a sensible weight successfully.

The value of being flexible but committed

A study carried out in Germany in 2003 monitored more than 1200 participants as they followed a long-term weight-reduction program. The study identified the behaviours that distinguished people who were successful in maintaining their weight loss over three years from those who were not. Success was defined as a weight loss of at least 5 per cent of initial weight as measured three years after the diet began. Results indicated that those who were successful had a flexible approach to eating and weight control. These people:

- achieved a basic shift in their dietary lifestyle but allowed occasional transgressions
- avoided snacking and nibbling but ate three meals a day
- tended to avoid doing other activities as they ate and to eat fruit and vegetables in preference to high-fat and high-sugar foods, and
- had integrated physical activity into their everyday lives and could deal with stress adaptively.

If you binge occasionally, it is important to find a strategy to deal with this problem. People who binge-eat tend to have a history of weight-cycling, in which they have gone on and off diets regularly. Binge-eating should not be confused with the dietary 'lapses' that everyone has, regardless of their weight-loss success. Binge-eating is often emotional eating. If your eating is a mechanism for coping with anxiety, depression or sadness, you could have a problem with stress management. See page 44 for more on dealing with stress.

4 Watch and record what you do

Earlier we talked about the importance of setting yourself dietary and exercise goals you can commit to, and of establishing a plan for achieving your goals. A critical component of success is to maintain a record of your advances towards your goals. You could keep a notebook in which you record your food and drink intake each day, together with your exercise activity. Weighing yourself regularly also provides important feedback, although you should be careful not to weigh yourself too regularly (see page 18). You might also want to share your achievements with others on a regular basis.

Although it is critical to be consistent in recording your behaviour, you should not use what you write as a reason to give up on your diet or exercise plans when things don't go exactly to plan. Failing to achieve a goal indicates the need for renewed commitment, but should never be used as an excuse for giving up.

5 Anticipate challenges and plan to overcome them

You will inevitably face many challenges and setbacks on your path to a new lifestyle, but recognising and accepting this in advance will help you plan to minimise these challenges. As far as possible, use your friends and family as social support so that they can help you acknowledge your success and keep any setbacks in perspective. Be prepared for the fact that stressful life events may make it more difficult for you to stick with your healthy regimen. Research indicates that regaining weight is often associated with stress, whereas people who successfully maintain weight loss report stable circumstances. Because we all experience stress, good social support – from weight-loss or exercise groups, or from family and friends – is helpful in maintaining a healthy lifestyle in the long term.

The way people react to stress is reflected in their coping strategies. Some people who regain weight have a coping style that leads them to eat in response to negative emotions or life events. People who are successful at maintaining weight loss are generally those who cope actively and directly with stressors. They find a solution to their problem or look for a healthy activity to replace the unhealthy activity they may have turned to in the past. A problem-solving approach to challenges enables us to treat negative experiences as setbacks to be overcome rather than excuses for giving up. Seeking help from family, friends or a professional counsellor is important if you are experiencing difficulties.

6 Recognise situations that are risky for you

Part of your plan for achieving a healthy lifestyle involves recognising the challenges that apply particularly to you. For example, you may belong to a social group that goes out for drinks and a meal after work every Friday and regularly have too much to eat or drink on these

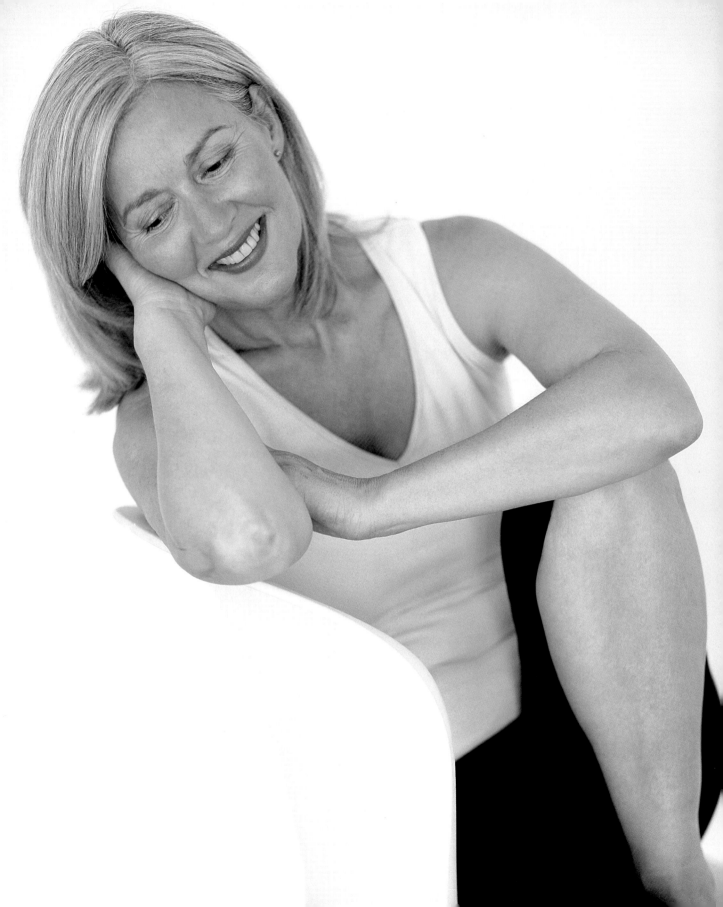

occasions. Or you may be a committed chocolate-eater who finds it difficult to pass a confectionery display without buying something. Or you may like to eat snack foods while you watch TV. Perhaps your partner drinks nothing but sugary soft drinks and this is a constant temptation for you.

Your goal must be to identify your risky situations and develop a strategy for coping with them. This may involve avoiding the situation altogether, substituting alternative behaviours, or enlisting social support. For example, you could enlist the help of your work colleagues on Friday-night outings to minimise your exposure to temptation. You could do this by substituting a glass of water for alcoholic drinks on alternate rounds and choosing restaurants with healthier options. If you are a chocolate-lover you should find a way to indulge your craving only moderately, and if you are addicted to snacking while you watch TV, you could consider snacking on healthier foods. If you're having trouble because your partner drinks soft drinks all the time, you could explain your issues to them and ask them to help you avoid temptation.

Although risky situations do vary from person to person, some experiences do often lead to a risk of over eating or choosing unhealthy foods. These include feeling hungry, sad, depressed, stressed or nervous; being at a social gathering with others; watching TV; or when food is relatively easily available, for example, at a buffet or party or when you are grocery shopping.

7   Maintain the right attitude

As we have seen, success in achieving lifestyle changes in the long term is critically dependent upon your attitude to the challenge. Success involves more than simply eliminating certain foods from your diet. It involves committing to a healthy eating and exercise plan that will make you look good, feel better and live longer. It also involves realising at the outset that you will encounter challenges, but deciding that you are prepared to deal with these using active problem-solving.

How do you get the right attitude? The strategies we have outlined here are designed to help you understand, predict and control critically important aspects of your life. Each is designed to address a particular purpose or overcome a particular challenge. And so each will make an important contribution to maintaining a good attitude and achieving your goals.

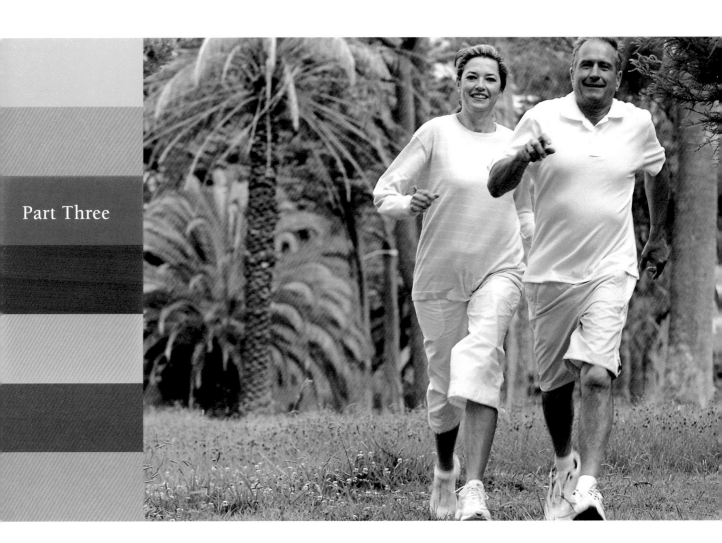

Part Three

The CLIP exercise program

by Dr Grant Brinkworth

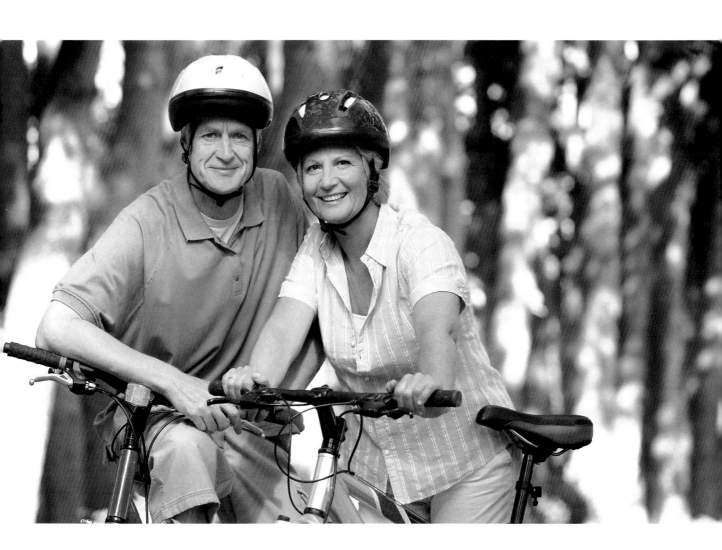

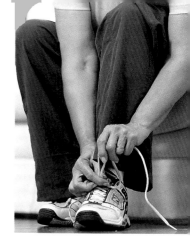

First things first

If you have decided to start an exercise program, you are already on your way to a healthier heart and a fitter body.

The first step you should take is to see your doctor, especially if any of the following applies to you.

- You are taking a prescription medicine.
- You have ever had any kind of heart problem.
- You have type 2 diabetes.
- You have problems with your bones or joints.
- You have high blood pressure and do not take medication for it.
- You have a family history of heart disease or stroke.
- You are a man over 35 or a woman over 40 and you are not used to doing even moderate levels of exercise.
- You are a smoker.
- You are very overweight or obese.

Your doctor will advise you on the best approach to take for exercise and what you should look out for.

Staying motivated

The hardest thing with starting a new exercise program is to stay motivated. Everybody loses interest in exercising from time to time, but this is often simply because their routine lacks variety. The key is to know how to respond to this challenge. Here are some ways to increase the variety of your exercise and your motivation to do it.

1 **Exercise with a partner**
   People who exercise with a partner almost always stick to their routine for longer. Choose someone who has similar goals and a similar fitness level to yours and make a commitment to each other to show up for every workout. Your partner will keep you motivated, push you to do more than you would on your own, and may also help you stay on track with your eating plan.

2 Use exercise videos

The biggest problem with exercise videos is that most people who buy them never end up using them, but they can be a great way to add variety to your exercise program. If you don't want to purchase your own, you can always borrow them from your local library. Try swapping one day of your own program for a home-exercise video workout every once in a while.

3 Take a class

If you've been doing your home-based exercise program, mix it up by taking an occasional exercise class at your local gym or leisure centre. A class adds the extra motivation of an instructor, upbeat music, variety, group support and a specific exercise time to keep you on track.

4 Do the opposite

If you've been doing your muscle-strengthening exercise with a whole-body routine, break your workouts up into upper body and lower body or change the order in which you do the exercises. You could also combine your aerobic exercise and muscle-strengthening exercises in the same workout by doing half of each at each workout. If you're bored with your muscle-strengthening routine, then simply change some of the exercises for new ones. Changing your routine for just one week can make a big difference to your enthusiasm. You might even find that you like the new routine better than your old one.

Your exercise diary

An exercise diary will help you maintain a detailed record of your workouts and keep track of your progress so that you can make every workout really count. Your exercise diary should record not only which exercises you have done, but also your thoughts and feelings before and after your workouts. Were you tired before you exercised? Did you run out of energy halfway through? How did you feel afterwards? Were you frustrated by your training session? Were you bored with the exercise? These are extremely important aspects to document when keeping your exercise diary, and will allow you to adjust your program so that it keeps working for you and you are less likely to get bored.

A sample exercise diary is given in Appendix 2, pages 259–60.

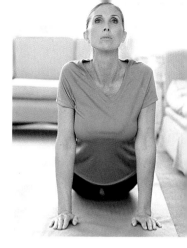

Warm-up, stretch and cool-down

Whenever you do any exercise, whether it is muscle-strengthening or aerobic exercise, you should make sure you warm up before you start, cool down after you finish, and stretch before and after.

1 Warm-up (10–15 minutes)

Too often, people don't warm up before exercising. In your warm-up you should lightly use the muscles you'll be targeting during your exercise. This will ensure that your muscles have an adequate supply of blood and will increase muscle temperature.

An ideal warm-up is light cardiovascular exercise that increases your breathing and heart rate (such as walking or jogging, or jogging on the spot) followed by stretching the key muscle groups to be worked during the main exercise – for example, calves, hamstrings, quadriceps and inner thighs for brisk walking. See page 62 for some good stretching exercises. You should warm up for at least 10 minutes.

2 Cool-down (10–15 minutes)

A proper cool-down is just as essential as a good warm-up. It will help you bring your heart rate and breathing back to normal and prevent the blood pooling in your exercising muscles, which can cause light-headedness or fainting. This will also help remove waste products from muscles. The most popular form of cool-down is light walking followed by stretching. Cooling down for a minimum of 10 minutes is a good option.

You should always incorporate stretches into your cool-down. They may help you avoid post-workout muscle stiffness and cramping.

3 Stretching

Stretch slowly and gently, and always breathe during stretching – never hold your breath. Hold each stretch for 10–30 seconds. The pages that follow give suitable stretches for each of the muscle groups you will be working, either in your walking program or your muscle-strengthening program.

Stretching exercises

These stretching exercises are for use as part of your warm-up, to prepare your muscles for the exercise to come, and as part of your cool-down, to reduce muscle stiffness.

- Only perform stretches after you have done a light warm-up (see page 61).
- Do not bounce, and always stretch only to the point of mild tension, without discomfort. If you overstretch you may cause damage. Back off if the stretch feels painful.

- Do not hold your breath during the stretches. Breathe slowly and naturally.
- Hold each stretch for 10–30 seconds and repeat 2–3 times.

Lower-body stretches

Calves

1 Lean against a wall with your forearms or palms.

2 Place your left leg straight back behind you, with your heel firmly planted on the floor, your right leg bent and your right foot about halfway between your left foot and the wall.

3 Starting with your back straight, gradually move your hips forward and

bend the knee of your right leg until you feel a stretch in the calf muscle of your left leg. Keep your left heel flat, your toes pointing straight ahead and your hips and shoulders parallel to the wall.

4 Hold, relax, then repeat the stretch with your right leg behind you.

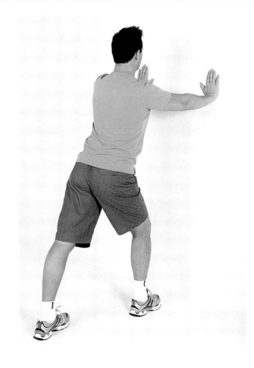

Hamstrings

1. Sit on the floor with both legs straight out in front of you.

2. Bend your left leg and place your left foot beside your right knee.

3. Keeping your left leg relaxed, your back straight and your head facing forwards, slowly bend at the hips (not waist) towards your right foot, until you feel a stretch in your right leg.

4. Hold, relax, then repeat with your right leg bent.

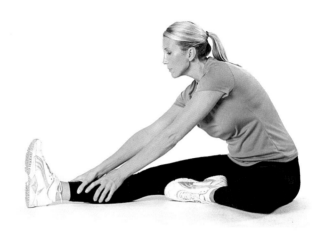

Quadriceps

1. Lie on your left side with your knees together.

2. Contract your abdominal muscles and, keeping your left leg straight, bend your right leg, grasping your right foot with your right hand. If you can't reach your foot comfortably, wrap a towel or belt around it and grasp this.

3. Slowly pull your right foot towards your right buttock, while slowly pushing your pelvis forward, until you feel a stretch in your right upper thigh.

4. Hold, relax, then repeat, lying on your right side.

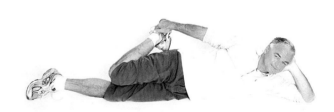

Inner thighs

1 Stand up straight with your feet slightly pointed out and a little more than hip-width apart. If necessary, hold on to something (such as the back of a chair) for balance.

2 Keeping your left leg straight, bend the knee of your right leg, moving your hip towards your right knee and leaning to the right.

3 Hold, relax, then repeat, leaning to the left.

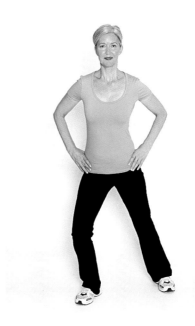

Upper-body stretches

Upper back

1 Stand up straight with your feet hip-width apart and your knees slightly bent.

2 Interlock your fingers and turn your palms out.

3 Keeping your body upright, extend your arms out in front of you at shoulder height until you feel a stretch between your shoulder blades.

4 Hold, relax and repeat.

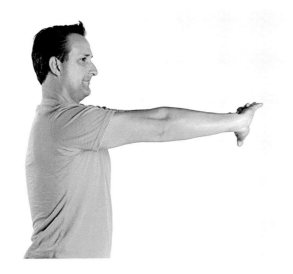

Shoulders and back of upper arm

1 Stand up straight with your feet hip-width apart.

2 Bring your right arm straight across your chest towards your left shoulder.

3 Keeping your upper body stable, use your left arm to ease your right elbow across your chest towards your left shoulder.

4 Hold, relax, then repeat, stretching your left arm.

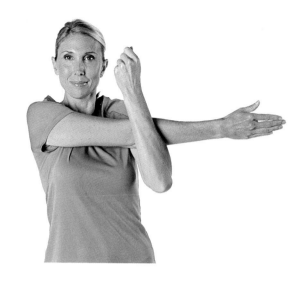

Shoulders

1 Stand up straight with your feet hip-width apart.

2 Interlock your fingers above your head with your palms facing upwards.

3 Push your hands further above your head as you exhale. You should feel the stretch in your shoulders.

4 Hold, relax and repeat.

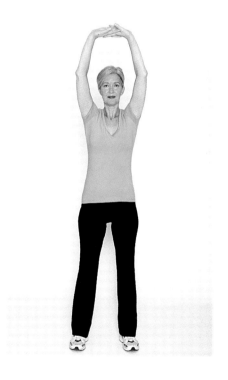

Chest

1 Stand up straight with your feet hip-width apart and your knees slightly bent.

2 With your arms behind you, interlock your fingers with your palms facing outwards.

3 Taking care not to lean forwards, stretch your arms back as far as possible, pulling back your shoulders and sticking out your chest. You should feel the stretch across your chest and in the front of your shoulders.

4 Hold, relax and repeat.

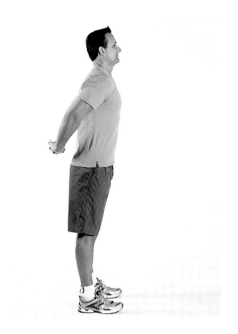

Triceps

1 Stand up straight with your feet hip-width apart and your knees slightly bent.

2 Place your left hand down the centre of your back, touching between your shoulder blades, with your fingers pointing downwards. Ensure your shoulders are relaxed.

3 Grasp your elbow with your right hand and push down on it gently, aiming to push your fingers down your spine.

4 Hold, relax, then repeat, stretching your right arm down your back.

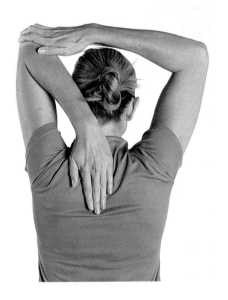

Sides

1 Stand up straight with your feet slightly more than hip-width apart and your knees slightly bent.

2 Lift your left arm above your head, with your left elbow bent and your left hand over your head.

3 Taking care not to lean forwards or backwards, slowly bend to the right at your waist, reaching your left arm over and across until you feel a stretch in your left side.

4 Hold, return to an upright position, then repeat with your right arm above your head.

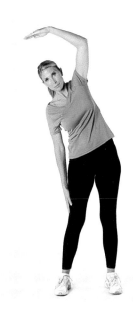

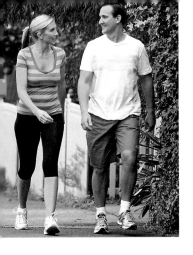

Walking program

There are many ways to begin an activity program. It should be based on regular, moderate- to vigorous-intensity aerobic exercise to improve your cardiovascular fitness, such as walking.

Aerobic activity uses large muscle groups, can be maintained for extended periods in a rhythmic fashion and makes your heart and lungs work harder. This will not only significantly reduce your risk of CVD and make you feel healthier, but also promote the greatest energy expenditure and have the biggest impact on weight control.

Walking and jogging are great forms of aerobic exercise that give your large muscle groups a good workout. They are also good for your heart, and will reduce the risk of chronic diseases such as CVD. Walking is simple, inexpensive, requires no special talent or athletic ability, can be done anywhere and places minimal stress on your body.

If your ability to walk or jog is limited by your weight, an injury or an orthopaedic problem (such as arthritis in your ankle, knee or hip), you may find non-weight-bearing exercise, such as swimming, cycling or rowing, more beneficial. These activities will provide similar health benefits without risking further discomfort or injury. If the exercise is fun, you are more likely to do it regularly and enjoy the resultant health benefits.

Your heart rate

Measuring your heart rate as you exercise is a great way to individualise your walking program. It also allows you to monitor how hard your aerobic exercise should be to ensure you achieve the greatest benefits from the program safely and effectively. If your heart rate is too low as you exercise, your body will reap little or no benefit from the activity. If it is too high, you will tire too quickly and run the risk of frustration, injury or giving up.

This technique not only allows you to measure your improvement easily, it also ensures that you are always working at the right level. As you become fitter, your average heart rate will decrease for the same amount of work. If you continued to walk at the same speed you would come to a point where the effort required would be much lower and so you would reap fewer benefits from your activity. By monitoring your heart rate and keeping it within desired zones, you can ensure that your health and fitness continue to improve.

You can work out what your heart rate (in beats per minute) should be during exercise by calculating your training heart rate (THR). Don't worry, it's easy! To determine your THR you must first determine your maximum heart rate (MHR) by subtracting your age from 220:

MHR = 220 minus age (in years)

example

Joe is 44 years old, so he can work out his MHR by subtracting 44 from 220:

MHR = 220 − 44 (years) = 176

So Joe's maximum heart rate would be 176 beats per minute.

Once you've calculated your maximum heart rate, you can calculate your training heart rate (THR) by taking a percentage of this value. Low-intensity exercise should give you a THR of 50–60 per cent of your MHR, higher-intensity exercise should give you a THR of 75–85 per cent of your MHR.

example

Say Joe wants to start an exercise program with a low-intensity aerobic activity. His heart rate as he exercises (THR) should be 50 per cent of his maximum heart rate of 176 beats per minute. He can calculate this percentage by dividing 176 by 100 and multiplying the answer by 50:

THR = 176 ÷ 100 × 50 = 88 beats per minute

When beginning your exercise program, particularly if you have not been active for a long time, it is best to start at a low intensity and increase gradually to the upper end of the range over time. As a general rule, you should exercise at an intensity between 65 and 85 per cent of your maximum heart rate.

example

Joe has been exercising regularly for a while and feels his improvements are beginning to plateau. He needs to increase his training heart rate (THR), and wants to move to 75 per cent of his maximum heart rate. He can calculate his new THR by dividing his MHR, 176 beats per minute, by 100 and multiplying by 75:

THR = 176 ÷ 100 × 75 = 132 beats per minute

For the 12-week walking program described here, you will first need to calculate three THR ranges (see 'Your three THR zones' below) for low, moderate and vigorous intensity. This will allow you to adapt your program as you become fitter.

Your three THR zones

Zone 1: Low intensity
For the beginner or people of low fitness

Your THR for Zone 1 should be 50–60 per cent of your MHR. For 50 per cent of MHR:

THR = MHR ÷ 100 × 50

We saw above that for Joe this figure is 88 beats per minute. For 60 per cent of MHR:

THR = MHR ÷ 100 × 60

For Joe, this calculation would be:

THR = 176 ÷ 100 × 60
= 106 beats per minute (rounded up)

So Joe's Zone 1 THR would be 88–106 beats per minute.

Zone 2: Moderate intensity

For people of average fitness

Your THR for Zone 2 should be 60–70 per cent of your MHR. We have already seen how to calculate 60 per cent of MHR. For 70 per cent of MHR:

$$THR = MHR \div 100 \times 70$$

For Joe this value would be:

$$THR = 176 \div 100 \times 70$$
$$= 123 \text{ beats per minute (rounded down)}$$

So Joe's Zone 2 THR would be 106–123 beats per minute.

Zone 3: Vigorous intensity

For people with a higher fitness level

For Zone 3, your THR should be 75–85 per cent of your MHR. For 75 per cent of MHR:

$$THR = MHR \div 100 \times 75$$

We have already seen that for Joe this value is 132 beats per minute. For 85 per cent of MHR:

$$THR = MHR \div 100 \times 85$$

For Joe this value would be:

$$THR = 176 \div 100 \times 85$$
$$= 150 \text{ beats per minute (rounded up)}$$

So Joe's Zone 3 THR would be 132–150 beats per minute.

By gradually increasing your intensity from Zone 1 to Zone 3, you will achieve greater improvements in your aerobic fitness. This will further reduce your risk of developing diabetes and CVD, and will enhance your health and wellbeing.

Here are a few things to bear in mind as you start your walking program.

- When doing aerobic exercise, you should never try to reach your THR immediately, because your muscles and circulatory system need to warm up slowly. Take it easy to begin with, and then slowly intensify your activity until you reach your THR.
- You should always go at your own pace, whatever your calculations might tell you. This is *your* program and it's important to increase the intensity of your walking program only when you feel comfortable doing so.
- If you can't complete your exercise in one continuous session, you can achieve similar health benefits by doing the same amount of exercise in several bouts of 10–15 minutes over the day. So instead of one continuous 45-minute walk, you might find it easier to do three 15-minute walks during the day.

Monitoring your heart rate

To stay within your THR zone during your training session, you will need to take your pulse periodically (see 'Determining your heart rate' opposite for instructions) as you are exercising. It is important to do this after at least 5 minutes of exercise, when your body has reached a steady state. Count the number of beats, always beginning with zero, for a ten-second period; then simply multiply this number by six and you have the number of heart beats per minute.

During an exercise session, Joe counts his pulse for ten seconds and finds it is 20. He can calculate his heart rate in beats per minute by multiplying this number by 6:

THR = 20 × 6 = 120 beats per minute

If your pulse is within your THR zone, you are on the right track and you can continue at that pace. If not, adjust your exercise intensity accordingly until you get into your zone. This may take some practice the first few times, but you will soon know how hard you need to be working and be able to estimate your heart rate with reasonable accuracy without having to monitor it regularly.

Determining your heart rate

There are several ways you can determine and monitor your heart rate and/or assess your exercise intensity as you exercise. Here are some of them.

1 Manual method

The most convenient place to measure the pulse is at the radial artery, which is located on the inside of your wrist, about 2 centimetres down from the base of your thumb. To measure your pulse, press firmly with the index and middle fingers of your other hand (do not use your thumb). If you are having trouble finding the pulse in your wrist, you could try the carotid pulse at the side of your neck, just under your jawbone. If you are taking your pulse at your neck, don't press too hard or your measurement will be inaccurate. Although the manual method is quick and convenient, it is sometimes difficult to use while you are exercising if you haven't had a lot of practice. Our heart rate during exercise correlates very closely with our heart rate during the early stages of recovery. This means that if you are having trouble monitoring your heart rate during exercise, you could monitor your exercise heart rate by stopping briefly, securing your pulse *immediately* after stopping and then counting the beats for 10 seconds. This will provide a reliable measure of your exercise heart rate.

2 Monitor method

An alternative is to use a heart-rate monitor. This may give you a more accurate heart-rate measurement, particularly during exercise, when your motion often makes it hard to get a clear manual measurement.

3 The talk-test method

The 'talk test' is a good subjective measure of your exercise intensity, and can be used in conjunction with your heart-rate measurement. When you are exercising at the desired intensity for cardiovascular health benefits, you should feel that the exercise is 'vigorous and challenging' but not 'strenuous'. You should still be able to talk comfortably with your exercise partner, but not be so comfortable that you can sing.

Note that if you are taking certain medications that affect heart rate, such as beta blockers, you may not be able to reach your THR. If this is the case, always obtain your doctor's approval before beginning any exercise program, and use the talk test to gauge your exercise intensity rather than taking your pulse.

The CLIP aerobic-fitness plan

A suggested 12-week walking program appears on page 259. The program is based on current exercise guidelines, the recommendations of leading health authorities and recent scientific research. It will be particularly useful if you are just beginning your exercise program, but if you have already been exercising for a while, you might need to increase your exercise intensity sooner.

This is only a suggested guide and you do not have to complete the whole program in 12 weeks. If you find a particular pattern tiring, repeat it before going on to the next. Listen to your body, and build the intensity and duration more slowly if you need to. Always proceed at your own pace.

Check your pulse periodically to see if you are exercising within your target THR zone. As you become fitter, try exercising within the upper range of your THR target zone and then move on to the next zone. Gradually increase the duration and frequency of your brisk walk from 30 to 60 minutes, and from 3 to 5 times a week. Although you can achieve significant health benefits by performing at least 30 minutes of moderate-intensity physical activity on five or more days a week, you will experience greater benefits to your fitness and health as you do more exercise more vigorously. Gradually increasing the duration of your exercise will help lower your risk of CVD and premature death further.

Although your goal is to achieve improvements in your health, you should also *enjoy* your activity. When you first start out, forget intensities, heart rates and THR zones. Just get out there and move. As your body starts to adjust, you can then start measuring and increasing the intensity and duration. Monitoring your exercise intensity is the best way to ensure you achieve the greatest benefit from the program safely and effectively.

You can also evaluate your aerobic fitness level by doing a simple test (see Appendix 1) at the start of and throughout your exercise program. This will allow you to see how much your fitness levels have improved.

Jogging

When you reach a level of fitness where you find you can no longer exercise at the appropriate intensity by walking, you can switch to jogging. You can do this gradually, by jogging part of the way and walking the rest, and then slowly build up to jogging the whole time. This will ensure you maintain your exercise intensity and enjoy maximum health benefits.

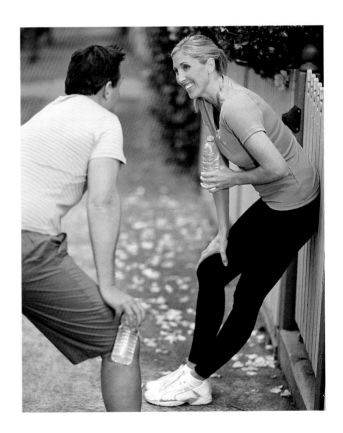

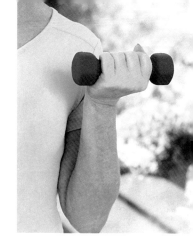

Muscle-strengthening program

People who lift weights or do any type of exercise that requires the body to work against a resistance are doing muscle-strengthening exercise.

This improves muscle strength and bone health, and research shows it also reduces the risk of chronic disease and premature death. Apart from promoting good health, it allows people to maintain their physical independence as they age.

Muscle-strengthening activities are an integral part of any health and fitness program for adults, regardless of their age or gender. Guidelines recommend that we do 8–10 muscle-strengthening exercises on at least two non-consecutive days each week. These exercises should use the major muscle groups, including the legs, arms, chest, back and stomach.

Many people think that you have to go to a gym to perform muscle-strengthening exercise, but an effective strength-training program actually takes only a few simple exercises. Best of all, they can be done at home, even while watching your favourite TV show. So no more excuses!

Muscle-strengthening plan

Most of the simple strength exercises in this program work the major muscle groups by using your body weight as resistance. Some also require dumbbells, inexpensive but handy pieces of equipment (see below). You can use the exercises as instructed, or you can use them to formulate your own program.

Wherever possible we have ensured that each muscle group has at least one exercise that can be performed entirely without equipment. This way, you can still do your exercise routine even when travelling.

Dumbbells

A dumbbell is a bar with weights on either end that is small enough to be held in one hand. These can either be of a set weight or allow for weight to be added or removed (see page 75). A barbell is much longer and designed to be used with both hands.

Dumbbells are remarkably versatile and useful tools for exercise and weight management. Pretty much everything you can do with fancy machines at the gym you can do at home with a simple dumb-bell set. These sets are relatively cheap and readily available in a variety of shops and sports stores.

We have grouped the exercises in terms of which muscle group they predominantly work. The major muscle areas and the muscle groups you will need to work are as follows.

- Upper body
  * Shoulders*
  * Chest*
  * Upper back*
  * Triceps⁺
  * Biceps⁺
- Core
  * Abdominals*
  * Lower back*
- Lower body
  * Buttocks*
  * Upper leg*
  * Lower leg⁺

You must include at least one exercise for the muscle groups marked with an asterisk (*). Exercises for muscle sets marked with a plus (⁺) are 'free choice' – include them if you want to.

For your exercise routine, you should select nine exercises that suit you from those recommended in the following pages. As indicated above, for the upper body you *must* include exercises for the shoulders, upper back and chest. You can also add the optional exercises for the biceps or triceps if you wish. For the core, you *must* include exercises for both the abdominals and the lower back. And for the lower body, you *must* include exercises for the buttocks and upper legs, and you can also add the optional lower leg exercise if you wish. Where appropriate, we have given a beginner, intermediate and advanced version of each exercise so that you can modify your program as you become stronger.

The nine exercises you select should form the basis of your muscle-strengthening program. If you wish, you can add one more to make ten, but you should avoid adding too many more. This is because overtraining can limit your results and lead to injury. And remember, if you get bored with your routine, just change it.

Perform your routine at least twice a week on non-consecutive days, completing 2–3 sets of 10–15 repetitions for each exercise (see 'Reps and sets' below). This will complement your aerobic walking program. Alternate your aerobic walking program and your muscle-strengthening program from day to day when you first start.

Reps and sets

A *rep* (repetition) is one complete action of the exercise involved. For example, for a biceps curl, one complete repetition would involve lifting the dumb-bell up and then lowering it again. If you want to do 10 reps, you need to perform the action ten times in a row without stopping.

This group of reps forms one *set*. For example, if you want to perform 2 sets of 10 reps, you need to repeat the exercise 10 times, have a short break, and then repeat the exercise 10 more times.

If an exercise involves one arm or one leg and you are required to complete 10 reps, this *does not* mean 5 reps for each arm or leg – 10 reps mean that you must complete the movement 10 times with each arm or leg.

Program instructions

Here are some requirements, suggestions and strategies for achieving success with this program.

1 Use the correct weights

For the exercises that require dumbbells, make sure you use the right dumbbell weights. If they are too light, you will gain no benefit from lifting them, but if they're too heavy, you will risk injuring yourself. To determine which is the right starting weight for you, try completing 10–15 repetitions in one set. If you can do it too easily, go up a notch; if you cannot get through the reps, try a lighter weight. Make sure you have a rest before you test the next size up or down.

Depending on the muscle involved and the exercise you're doing, you may need different weights for each exercise. If you use just one weight for every exercise you'll under-work some muscles and potentially strain or damage others. For this reason, it can be more useful to buy dumbbells with adjustable weights; as your fitness advances you can add supplementary weights without having to buy a whole new dumbbell.

When you can do 15 reps of an exercise easily, it is time to increase the weight you are lifting.

2 Use a mat

For some of the exercises you will need to lie on the floor, so buy an exercise mat or do the exercises on thick carpet to protect your back.

3 Check your posture

You must maintain the correct posture for each exercise to maximise strength gains and prevent injury.

4 Don't rush

Perform each exercise in a single, slow, controlled movement. Never jerk the weights or use too much force.

5 Take your time

Each phase of the exercise – the *lift* and the *return* phases – should take approximately 2 seconds to complete. For example, for a biceps curl, raising the weight to your shoulder should take 2 seconds, followed by a pause of 1 second, and then lowering the weight to its starting position should take another 2 seconds. Allow yourself a rest period of 1–2 minutes between each exercise set.

6 Breathe

Do not hold your breath during the movements. Remember to breathe *out* as you lift a weight and breathe *in* as you lower the weight back to the starting position.

7 Use correct technique

To avoid injury and gain the maximum benefit from your exercises, it's important to maintain correct weight-lifting technique at all times. Avoid 'cheating' – with many exercises you can 'cheat' by swinging your body and using momentum or other muscle groups to do the work. This is often tempting if you are struggling to achieve the final rep in a set, but avoid the temptation. Doing exercises incorrectly can result in sprains, torn muscles or other injuries. If you can't finish the last rep or set, despite your best efforts, that's fine. It's better to avoid injury, get the *maximum* benefit from the exercise and gradually improve rather than damage yourself just to reach a number. Avoid 'locking out' your joints – when performing the exercises, avoid extending your arms or legs until they are completely straight and your elbows or knees are 'locked'. Even when fully extending your arms or legs as part of an exercise you should keep a slight bend at your elbows and knees. Maintain a full range of motion – complete each exercise over the entire range of movement rather than doing only part of it. For example, when performing biceps curls, ensure that you flex your elbows fully and bring the dumbbell right up to your shoulder rather than stop halfway through the motion, which would limit the benefits of the exercise.

8 Keep an exercise diary

Keep a regular account of your exercise routines, recording the number of reps and sets you do, and record and monitor your heart rate for the aerobic walking program. See Appendix 2 (pages 259–60) for an exercise diary.

9 Drink water

Make sure you drink plenty of water before, during and after your exercise so that you remain adequately hydrated.

10 Wear comfortable clothing

Loose, comfortable clothing and supportive athletic shoes will keep you cool, protect you from injury and help keep you motivated.

Safety with dumbbells

Dumbbells are useful tools, but handling them without respect can result in injury. When picking up weights from the floor, make sure you *bend your knees* rather than use your back to lift them.

Some exercises with dumbbells require you to lie on the floor, which can make it awkward to pick the weight up without straining your shoulders. Here is a good procedure to adopt.

1 Sit on the floor with your feet on the floor and your knees bent at 45 degrees.
2 Pick up both dumbbells and hold them in front of your stomach or chest with the ends or 'heads' of the weights resting on your thighs.
3 Gently roll backwards until your back is on the floor. The dumbbells should now be resting gently on your chest.
4 Position your feet flat on the floor and you're in a great position to start your exercise.
5 Once you've finished a set, bring the weights back to your chest or stomach and roll back up into your initial sitting position.

It's also a good idea to run through each exercise without weights the first time you do it, until you're sure of exactly what you need to do.

Many shoulder exercises require you to extend your arms to the front and to the side. Before beginning any such exercise, ensure that there is sufficient space in the room for you to do this.

Lowering weights during an exercise and returning to your starting position can provide just as much benefit as raising them, so don't simply let your arms drop. Similarly, when raising weights, don't try to swing your arms up or you'll risk injury and the exercise won't provide any benefit.

Upper body
Shoulders

One-arm front deltoid raise

1 Stand with your feet hip-width apart, your back straight and your knees slightly bent.

2 Take a dumbbell in each hand. Hang your arms straight down in front of you, with your elbows slightly bent and your thumbs facing inwards.

3 Keeping your back straight, slowly raise your right arm until it is parallel with the ground. Pause, then slowly return your right arm to its starting position.

4 Repeat, raising your left arm.

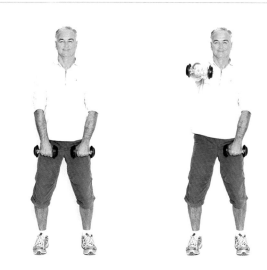

Lateral deltoid raise

1 Stand with your feet hip-width apart, your back straight and your knees slightly bent. Take a dumbbell in each hand and hang your arms by your sides with your palms facing inwards, taking care not to slouch.

2 Keeping your arms straight, slowly raise both until they are parallel with the floor and the backs of your hands are facing the ceiling. Your body should form a T shape. Pause, then slowly lower your arms to their starting position.

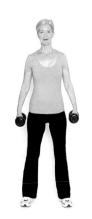
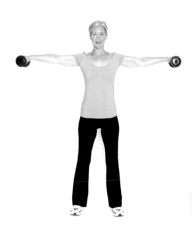

Overhead press

1 Sit on a stable chair or bench with your feet hip-width apart. Take a dumbbell in each hand and bend your elbows until your hands are just in front of and slightly to the side of your shoulders, your palms facing the front and your thumbs pointing inwards.

2 Keeping your back straight, slowly push the dumbbells straight up above your head, until your arms are almost straight but still slightly bent. Pause then slowly lower your arms to their starting position.

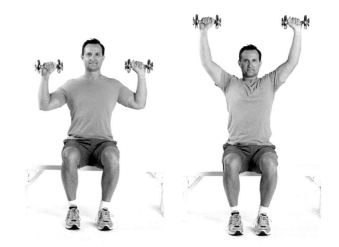

Chest

Push-up
Beginner

1 Stand facing a wall with your feet hip-width apart, then place your palms on the wall at shoulder height and slightly more than shoulder-width apart. Your arms should be almost straight but still slightly bent.

2 Keeping your back straight and using your arms to take your weight, slowly lean towards the wall until your nose almost touches it. Pause, then slowly push with your arms back to your starting position. Don't lock your elbows at the end of the movement; keep them slightly bent.

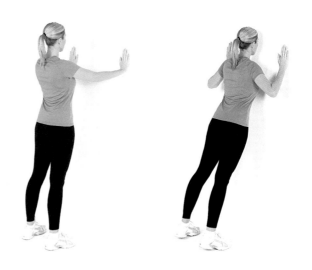

Intermediate/Advanced

1 Kneel on all fours with your back parallel with the floor. Your hands should be slightly more than shoulder-width apart and your elbows slightly bent.

2 Keeping your back straight, bend your elbows and slowly lower your body to the floor. Pause, then slowly push with your arms back to your starting position. Don't lock your elbows at the end of the movement. For Advanced, start with your legs straight out.

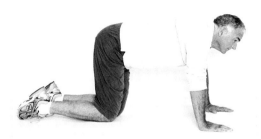

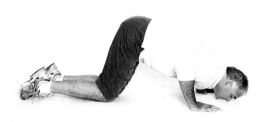

Chest fly with dumbbells

1 Lie on your back with your knees bent and your feet flat on the floor, hip-width apart. Take a dumbbell in each hand (see page 76) and stretch both arms out to your sides, with your elbows slightly bent and your palms facing upwards. Each arm should form a 90-degree angle with your body.

2 Keeping your elbows slightly bent throughout the movement, lift your arms straight up and bring them together until the dumbbells meet. Do not arch your back; this can cause injury and may mean you're trying to lift too much. Once your hands meet, pause, then slowly lower your arms to their starting position.

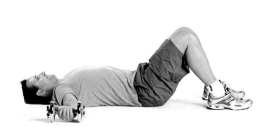

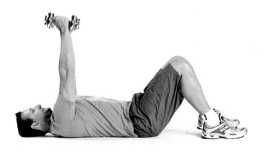

Upper back

Upright row

1 Stand with your feet slightly more than hip-width apart and your knees slightly bent. Take a dumbbell in each hand, and hang your arms straight down in front of your legs, with your palms facing inwards.

2 Taking care to keep your back straight and stable (focus on a spot high on the wall directly in front of you), your head up and your shoulders back, slowly 'row' the dumbbells up to your chest until your upper arms are parallel with the floor. Pause, then slowly return to your starting position.

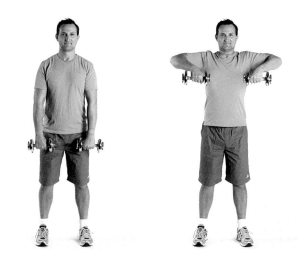

Bent-over row

1 Sit at the end of a flat bench or chair with your feet hip-width apart and lean forward so your chest almost touches your knees. Take a dumbbell in each hand and hang your arms straight down, with your palms facing inwards. Keep your head up and your shoulders back.

2 Keeping your elbows slightly bent, raise your arms straight out to the sides until they are parallel with the floor and the backs of your hands are pointing to the ceiling. Pause, trying to squeeze your shoulders together, then slowly return your arms to their starting position.

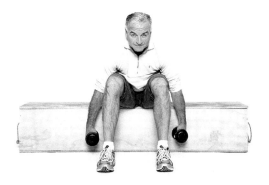 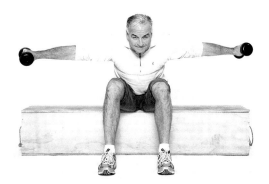

Triceps

Triceps dip
Beginner

1 Sit on the floor with your knees bent and your feet flat on the floor, hip-width apart. Put your hands just behind you, with your fingers pointing towards your body.

2 Keeping your back straight and your abdominal muscles tight, slowly and gently bend your elbows to about 90 degrees (no further) and lower your body towards the floor. Pause, then slowly return to your starting position.

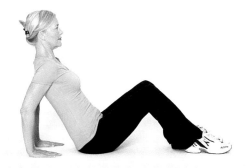

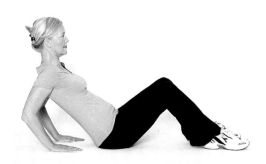

Intermediate/Advanced

1 Stand in front of a secure chair or stable surface of a similar height. Put your hands behind your back and on the chair, slightly more than shoulder-width apart. Walk your feet out until your knees are bent at 90 degrees and your upper legs are parallel with the floor, then lift your toes off the floor. Your arms should be almost straight but still slightly bent.

2 Keeping your back straight, your elbows in line with your hands and your legs relaxed, slowly lower your buttocks towards the floor until your upper arms are parallel with the ground. Pause, then use your hands (not your legs) to slowly push yourself back up to your starting position. For Advanced, walk your feet out until your legs are straight.

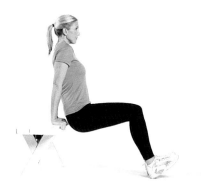

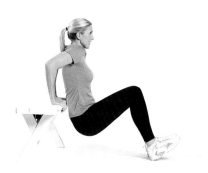

Standing triceps kickback with dumbbells

1 Stand up straight, with your feet hip-width apart. Take a dumbbell in each hand, bend your elbows and pull them in to your sides, with your hands near your shoulders and your palms facing your body. Bend your knees and lean forwards from the waist.

2 Keeping your back straight, your elbows tucked in and your upper arms still, straighten your arms by moving only your lower arms and extend them as far back as you can. Pause, then slowly return your arms to their starting position.

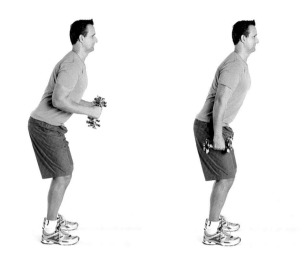

Biceps

Biceps curl

1 Sit on the edge of a bench or chair with your knees bent at 90 degrees, your feet flat on the floor and your back straight. Take a dumbbell in each hand and hang your arms by your sides with your palms facing towards your body.

2 Slowly bend your elbows and lift the dumbbells up towards your shoulders, twisting your lower arms as you go until your inner wrists face your biceps. Squeeze your biceps for 1 second, then slowly return your arms to their starting position.

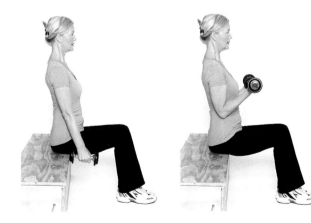

Hammer curl

1 Sit on the edge of a bench or chair with your knees bent at 90 degrees, your feet flat on the floor and your back straight. Take a dumbbell in each hand and hang your arms by your sides with your palms facing inwards, towards each other.

2 Slowly bend your elbows and lift the dumbbells up towards your shoulders while keeping your palms facing each other. Squeeze your biceps for 1 second, then slowly return your arms to their starting position.

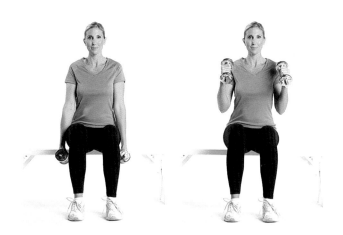

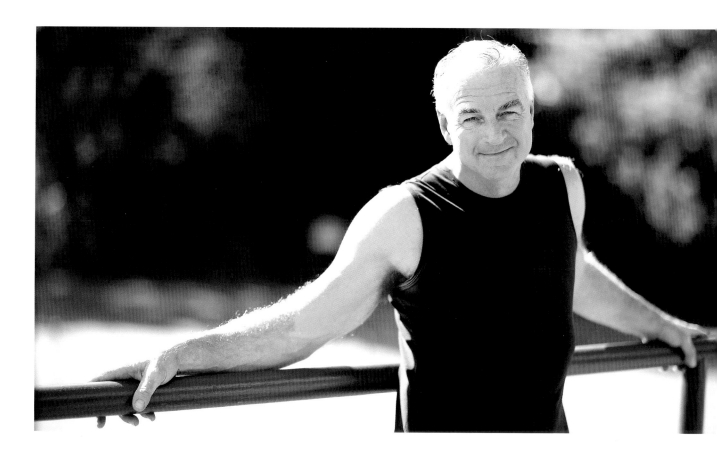

Core
Abdominals

Half crunch

1 Lie on your back with your knees bent and your feet flat on the floor. Ensure that your lower back is pushed down towards the floor. Cross your arms over your chest or place your hands lightly behind your head with your elbows out.

2 Leading with your chest, keeping your head and neck straight and ensuring that your motion comes from your abdominal muscles and is smooth throughout, lift your upper body off the floor, to an angle of no more than 30 degrees. Pause, then slowly uncurl to your starting position. Do not bend or pull your neck to lift your head off the floor. To increase the intensity of the exercise, hold your arms up straight above your head or hold a weight across your chest.

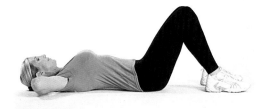 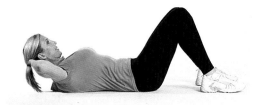

The plank

1 Lie on your tummy with your hands beside your shoulders and your feet together. To get into your starting position, keep your forearms and hands on the floor then bend your elbows to 90 degrees.

2 Relaxing your shoulders and bracing your abdominals, push up on your toes so that your legs are slightly off the floor and your body is parallel with the floor. Hold this position for 30 seconds, then return to your starting position.

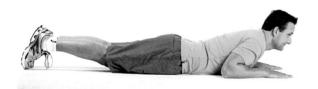

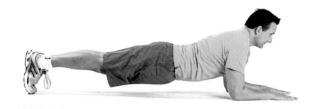

Lower back

Swim

1 Lie on your tummy with your arms stretched over your head, parallel with the floor, and your legs straight.

2 Slowly lift your right arm and your left leg towards the ceiling, as high as you can. Pause, then slowly lower your right arm and left leg back to their starting positions. Repeat, lifting your left arm and right leg.

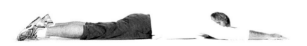

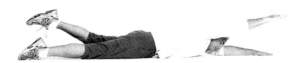

Lower body
Buttocks

Lying buttocks bridge

1 Lie on your back with your knees bent at 90 degrees and your feet flat on the floor. Place your arms by your sides with your palms flat on the ground.

2 Slowly raise your hips until your torso forms an angle of 45 degrees with the floor. Squeeze your buttocks together for 1 second, then slowly return to your starting position.

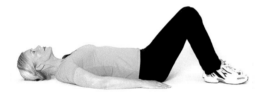

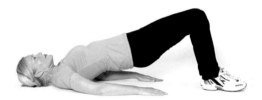

Glute kickback

1 Kneel on all fours with your back parallel with the floor.

2 Keeping your right knee at 90 degrees, slowly move your right foot back and up until your right thigh is parallel with the floor. Squeeze your buttocks for 1 second, then slowly return to your starting position. Repeat with your left leg.

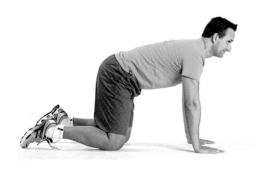

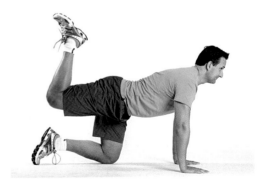

Upper leg

Squat
Beginner/Intermediate/Advanced

1 Stand up straight with your feet hip-width apart and your hands on your hips.

2 Keeping your back straight (focus on a spot high on the wall directly in front of you), slowly bend your knees and lower your body, until your thighs are almost parallel with the floor.

Try not to allow your knees to go further forward than your toes; if this happens, push your buttocks further back. Pause, then slowly return to your starting position. For Advanced, start with a dumbbell in each hand and your arms by your sides.

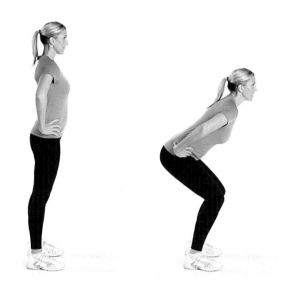

Lunge
Beginner/Intermediate/Advanced

1 Stand up straight with your hands on your hips and your feet hip-width apart.

2 Keeping your abdominal muscles tight and your back straight, take a good step back with your right leg and land on the ball of your right foot.

3 Still keeping your back straight, slowly bend your knees until your right knee is almost touching

the floor and your left thigh is parallel with the ground. Don't allow your left knee to go further forward than your left toe.

4 Pause, then return to your starting position.

5 Repeat with your left leg behind you. For Advanced, start with a dumbbell in each hand and your arms by your sides.

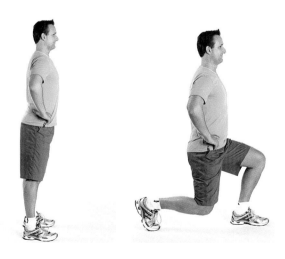

Step-up

Beginner/Intermediate/Advanced

1 Stand up straight beside a bench or a low, stable chair with your feet hip-width apart.

2 Keeping your back straight, step up onto the bench with your right foot, then lift your left foot so you are standing on the bench.

Pause, then leading with your right foot, carefully step back off the bench.

3 Repeat, leading with your left foot. For Advanced, start with a dumbbell in each hand and your arms by your side.

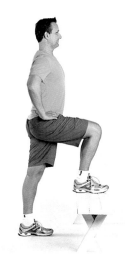 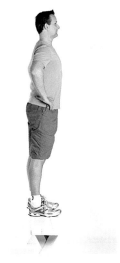

Lower leg

Calf raise

Beginner

1 Stand up straight with your feet hip-width apart.

2 Keeping your back straight, lift your heels as high as you can so that

you are on tiptoe. Pause, then slowly return to your starting position.

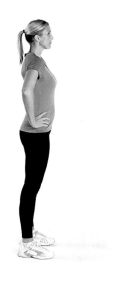 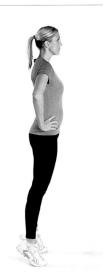

Intermediate/Advanced

1 Stand up straight with your feet hip-width apart.

2 Keeping your back straight, lift your right foot off the floor (let it hang, or rest it behind your left calf) then lift your left heel as high as you can so that you are on tiptoe. Pause, then slowly return to your starting position.

3 Repeat, lifting your left foot. For Advanced, start with a dumbbell in each hand and your arms by your side.

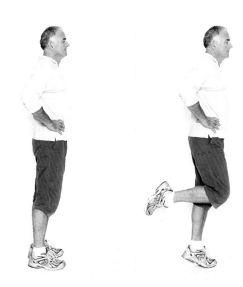

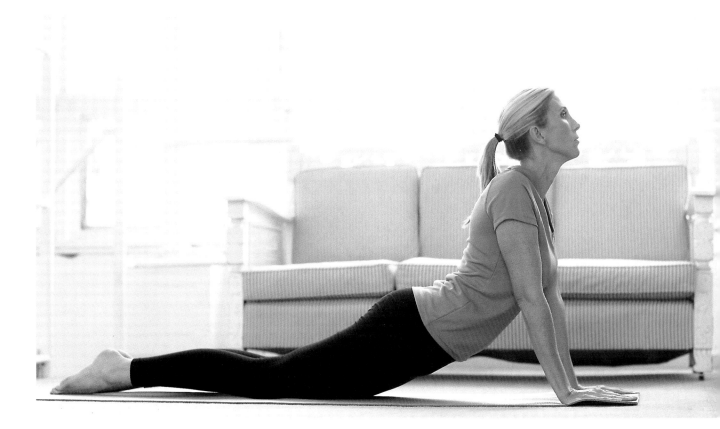

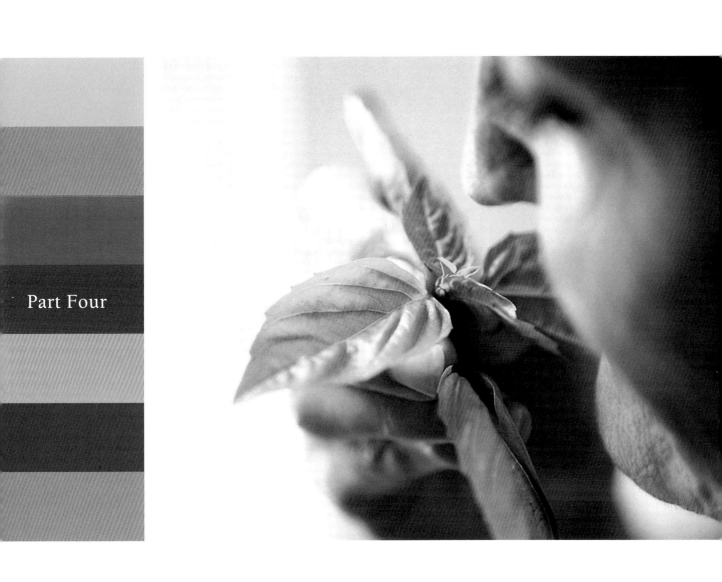

Part Four

Ten super CLIP foods

by Xenia Cleanthous, Gemma Williams,
Dr Manny Noakes, Dr Peter Nichols,
Dr Surinder Singh and Dr Mahinda Abeywardena

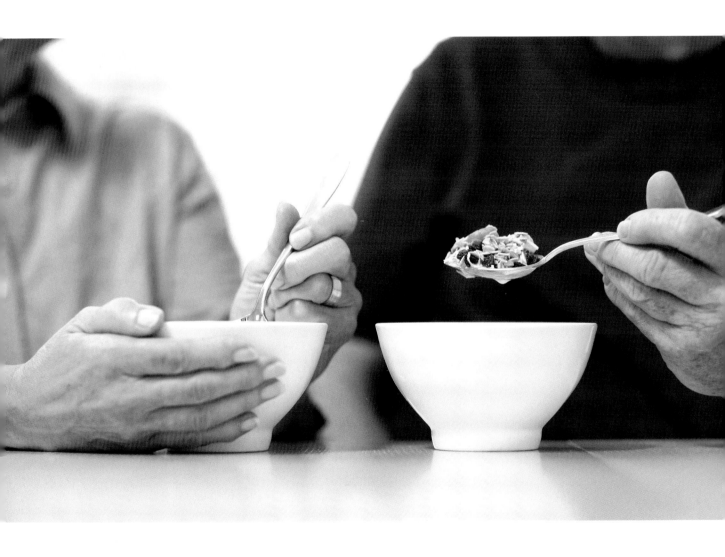

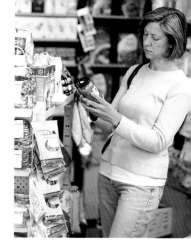

Good food for good health

The CLIP eating plan is nutritionally balanced and includes foods from all the food groups necessary for health and wellbeing. It also focuses on ten key foods that can have a positive impact on your cardiovascular health and cholesterol levels.

1 Fish and omega-3 fatty acids

The three omegas

Most people associate 'fats' with poor health, but our bodies do need some fats and, indeed, some are remarkably good for us, especially omega-3 fatty acids. Fatty acids are the main building blocks of most fats and oils. Omega-3 fatty acids occur in two main forms: long-chain, from marine sources, and shorter-chain. In this book and in CLIP we focus on the long-chain omega-3 fatty acids (which we will refer to as LC omega-3s from now on).

The health benefits of LC omega-3s

LC omega-3s are an essential fat, which means that the human body needs them to grow and function properly. Because the human body cannot produce its own LC omega-3s, and does not convert short-chain omega-3s to LC omega-3s very efficiently, we need to obtain LC omega-3s from dietary sources.

One of the most important health benefits of LC omega-3s is protection against CVD. In the mid-1980s,

CSIRO researchers first discovered that LC omega-3s can protect against death from heart attack by helping to maintain normal heart rhythm. These early observations have now been confirmed in some but not all human clinical trials. In the largest of these intervention trials, involving thousands of patients with heart disease, fish oil supplements reduced sudden cardiac death by half. The positive impact of LC omega-3s on our heart health includes:

- protection against death from heart attack by reducing the risk of abnormal heart rhythms
- lowering of high blood pressure (in high doses), and
- inhibiting the processes that lead to atherosclerosis.

LC omega-3s can also lower triglyceride levels by reducing their production in the liver. Indeed, purified LC omega-3s are now available for patients with very high triglyceride levels. LC omega-3s help combat some inflammatory conditions, such as rheumatoid arthritis. To achieve these benefits, however, requires large doses, so you should not attempt to self-medicate.

There is some preliminary evidence that LC omega-3s may be helpful for conditions such as Alzheimer's disease, dyslexia and attention deficit hyperactivity disorder (ADHD). They may also play a role in mood regulation and in maintaining good cognitive function as we age.

How we found out about LC omega-3s

The health benefits of LC omega-3s were first noticed about three decades ago. Scientists observed that Greenland Inuit had lower rates of heart disease than other ethnic groups, despite the fact their diet is traditionally high in fat. They also found that Inuit blood took longer to clot. It was found that the traditional, seafood-rich diet of the Inuit was responsible both for their thinner blood and healthier hearts. The key nutrient in this diet was LC omega-3s.

Suggested omega-3 intakes

The recommended daily intake of LC omega-3s for Australians is about 500 milligrams. The current average intake in Australia, the United Kingdom and the United States is estimated to be only 100–200 milligrams a day. This is not enough if we are to combat heart disease and other chronic disorders. To obtain sufficient amounts of LC omega-3s, we suggest at least 2 meals of oily fish a week at both lunch and dinner. This amount is provided by the CLIP eating plan. The processing and cooking of seafood won't damage LC omega-3s, but always avoid deep-frying your food. For people with heart disease, a 1 gram fish oil supplement each day is recommended.

Animal sources of LC omega-3s

The main source of LC omega-3s is seafood, including fish, lobsters, oysters and squid. Some animal foods such as lean red meat and eggs contain LC omega-3s, but in smaller quantities than fish. Land plants, such as canola and linseed, do contain some omega-3s but they are shorter-chain varieties. These are beneficial, but do not provide the same health benefits as LC omega-3s.

Most fish is low in kilojoules, which makes it a particularly good option when eating out. The trick is to make sure you choose healthy cooking options, such as grilling, poaching, baking or steaming. Avoid battered, fried or crumbed seafood, which are likely to be high in saturated fats and kilojoules. Although you can take fish oil supplements to obtain your recommended intake of omega-3s, you'll be missing out on the additional nutrients that seafood contains.

Different types of fish contain different amounts of LC omega-3s. White-fleshed Australian wild fish, for example, contain on average approximately 350 milligrams of LC omega-3s per 150 grams (a typical serving size). The same amount of slender tuna, however, contains 5640 milligrams and swordfish 1530 milligrams.

Even different parts of the same fish can contain different amounts of LC omega-3s. The season and location in which a fish was caught can also make a difference, although these are usually only minor variations. CSIRO has a particular interest in LC omega-3s and, in partnership with the Fisheries Research and Development Corporation, has profiled the LC omega-3 content of a range of wild and farmed seafood and of other protein foods.

Australian farmed fish can have up to ten times the concentration of LC omega-3s of fish caught in the wild. This depends, however, on the type of diet the farmed fish eat. If they are fed fishmeal or fish oil, the LC omega-3 concentrations will be high, but if not, they will have much lower LC omega-3 levels.

The pressures on wild fish stocks are increasing, and the numbers of large fish in the oceans are only

10 per cent those of pre-industrial times. We therefore require alternative ways to supply enough LC omega-3s to maintain human health. The research of the CSIRO Food Futures Flagship is now focused on developing land plants with LC omega-3s. We hope that in the next few years people will be able to obtain these healthy fats from plants rather than fish.

How safe is my snapper?

The levels of mercury in most fish caught and sold in Australia are low. It is important for young children, pregnant or breastfeeding women and women who are planning to conceive to limit their intake of some species – shark (flake), broadbill, marlin, swordfish, orange roughy (also sold as deep-sea perch) and catfish. Many people mistake these warnings about excessive consumption of large fish for a warning against *all* fish. The mercury issue has at times also been overstated; seafood also contains selenium, which counteracts the effects of mercury. For information on fish and mercury levels, visit the Food Standards Australia New Zealand website, www.foodstandards.gov.au/foodmatters/mercuryin fish.cfm.

Plant sources of omega-3s

Some plant foods are good sources of shorter-chain omega-3 fatty acids, such as alpha-linolenic acid (ALA). These include flaxseed, canola, walnut and soybean oils. ALA is an essential fat. Although studies have shown an association between high ALA intake and lower rates of death from heart attack, ALA has not been tested for its effect on the rate of heart attack. The evidence for any benefit of ALA on heart attack rates is lower and less consistent than the effect of LC omega-3s from fish. Plant omega-3 fats are important, and CLIP includes them.

2   Soluble fibre

Dietary fibre occurs in all cereal foods, legumes, fruit and vegetables. The two main types are soluble and insoluble fibre, which work together to help keep your digestive system healthy. Soluble fibre can also help reduce your blood cholesterol levels. It is thought to do this by holding on to the cholesterol and bile acids (which are made from cholesterol) and removing them from your body, thus preventing the cholesterol from being absorbed.

Oat-based cereals, barley, psyllium-enriched cereals and linseed are all excellent sources of soluble fibre, as are fruit, vegetables, legumes and soy products. The CLIP eating plan includes plenty of these foods, so you're sure to get your soluble fibre needs each day.

3   Low-fat dairy foods

Dairy foods are a major source in our diet of calcium, which is important for bone health. They also provide a valuable source of protein, which is important for maintaining our muscle tissue as well as in controlling our appetite. Full-fat dairy products, such as butter, cream, cheese and whole milk, however, contain mostly saturated fats. This means that they can increase our LDL cholesterol levels if we eat them in large quantities and on a daily basis.

Low-fat dairy foods are preferable, as they still provide valuable calcium and protein but are much lower in saturated fat. The CLIP eating plan recommends 2–3 serves of low-fat dairy foods each day. Full-fat cheese is limited to twice a week, and soft margarines and oils are included in preference to butter.

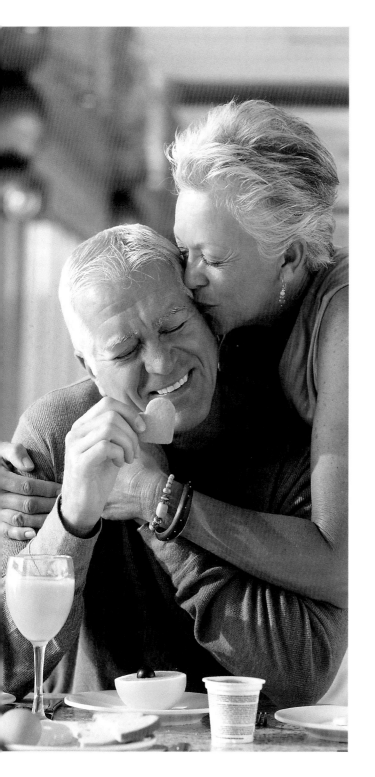

4 Nuts

Nuts are an excellent source of protein and many other nutrients essential for good health. They are generally high in healthy monounsaturated and polyunsaturated fats, and low in saturated fat. They also contain fibre, folate, arginine, plant sterols and antioxidants such as vitamin E, all of which contribute to optimum health. People who regularly consume nuts have a reduced risk of CVD, which is thought to be due to a lowering of LDL cholesterol levels and the maintenance of healthy blood vessels.

The best nuts

A good variety of nuts in the right amounts is the way to go. Tree nuts, including almonds, Brazil nuts, cashews, hazelnuts, macadamias, pecans and walnuts are all suitable. Peanuts are technically a legume, but their nutrient profile is so similar to other nuts that they are included in this category. Although chestnuts are classified as nuts, they are much higher in carbohydrate and lower in fat and protein than most nuts, so eat these less often. You should limit the coconut and palm nuts you eat, as these contain large amounts of saturated fats. Always choose dry-roasted, unsalted nuts. Walnuts are especially high in shorter-chain plant omega-3s, so you may like to eat these more often.

Serving sizes

Nuts are packed with nutrients but they do contain a lot of kilojoules, so we need to be careful about the quantity we eat. A good handful of nuts each day is a great alternative to high-saturated-fat processed snack foods. The CLIP eating plan includes 20 grams of raw, unsalted nuts each day.

5 Legumes

Also known as pulses, this group of plant foods includes peas, beans and lentils. Legumes are an excellent source of fibre and soluble fibre (see page 95). They are also a great low-fat, low-GI source of carbohydrates, as well as many other nutrients vital to wellbeing, including iron, calcium, zinc and B-group vitamins.

They provide an excellent, affordable vegetarian protein option and are available tinned or dried. The most common tinned varieties include chickpeas, kidney beans, baked beans and bean mixes; always choose salt-reduced options. Legumes such as split peas, soybeans and lentils are more commonly available dried; they need to be soaked overnight before cooking.

In line with recommendations from the Heart Foundation, the CLIP menu plans (see page 124) include at least two legume meals (lunch or dinner) each week. Legumes can be exchanged for other carbohydrate sources in your diet (see page 106) or for protein sources. Add them to soups, stir-fries, casseroles or salads, or make them into patties.

6 Whole grains

Whole grains are cereal foods that still contain all three components of the natural grain: the endosperm (the main part), the germ (the smallest part) and the bran (the outer layer). The grain can be intact or processed – milled or cracked, for example. Whole grains include wheat, oats, rice, rye, barley and corn.

Wholegrain foods are an excellent source of carbohydrate, fibre, iron and the B-group vitamins. Research shows wholegrain foods can reduce the risk of CVD. This is thought to be due to the combination of key nutrients they contain, including fibre, magnesium, vitamin E, folate and vitamin B6. In contrast, refined cereal foods, which are low in fibre, are associated with a higher body weight and a higher risk of CVD.

Being high in fibre, especially insoluble fibre (fibre that does not dissolve in water), wholegrain foods encourage good bowel health. Insoluble fibre helps prevent constipation and promotes regular bowel function. Whole grains also provide indigestible carbohydrate, which promotes the growth of healthy bacteria in the large intestine.

Wholegrain foods provide many other health benefits. They have been linked to lower risk of type 2 diabetes, and to improved bowel health.

The most common wholegrain foods include wholegrain (multigrain) bread, crisp breads and rice cakes, wholegrain breakfast cereals, brown rice and couscous. Wholemeal bread and pasta, and other products made with wholemeal flour, are great carbohydrate options. Foods made with white flour provide far fewer health benefits than their wholegrain counterparts. This is because white flour is refined to remove the outer layers of the grain (the bran and germ), where most of the nutrients are found. The same is true for white rice.

Eating refined-grain foods rather than wholegrain foods can also increase blood triglyceride levels. Triglyceride levels are also increased by eating *large* amounts of foods containing fructose, such as fruit, dried fruit and fruit juices, and by gaining weight. CLIP can lower triglycerides very effectively because it is high in whole grains and low in refined-carbohydrate foods.

How much is enough?
A daily intake of at least 6 grams of wholegrain fibre is a good minimum target to aim for. In food terms this is equal to about 100 grams (2½ slices) of wholegrain

bread. The CLIP eating plan has been designed to include 2 slices of wholegrain bread and 40 grams of high-fibre breakfast cereal each day, which will ensure you obtain enough wholegrain fibre.

A total daily fibre intake of 25–30 grams or more will help keep your digestive system healthy. By combining wholegrain foods with fruit, vegetables and other carbohydrate options, we have ensured that the CLIP eating plan provides around 35 grams of soluble and insoluble fibre in total – more than enough to meet your daily needs.

7   Alcohol

Alcoholic drinks are widely enjoyed throughout society, and research shows that in moderate amounts they can benefit heart health, especially in older people. This is because alcohol increases the level of protective HDL cholesterol in the blood. The protective effects seem to come from the alcohol itself rather than from antioxidants or compounds found in the drinks. Those who drink moderate amounts of alcohol have been shown to have a lower risk of CVD and to live longer than teetotallers or those who drink more than they should (more than 2 standard drinks a day).

It is important to remember that alcohol is still a source of kilojoules, which should give you an added incentive to drink only in moderation. If you do not drink, then we are not recommending that you start. And if you do drink, there is no reason to increase your alcohol intake if you are currently drinking less than the guidelines. The guidelines for safe drinking are:
- 2 standard drinks a day for men (maximum 6 a day)
- 1 standard drink a day for women (maximum 4 a day)
- 1–2 alcohol-free days a week for men and women.

The CLIP eating plan allows up to 6 standard drinks a week, which is well within these guidelines.

What is a standard drink?
One standard drink is the amount of that drink that contains 10 grams of alcohol. Depending on the strength of the alcoholic drink, 1 standard drink can vary in volume quite considerably. One standard drink is equal to:
- 200 millilitres regular beer
  (4.9 per cent alcohol content)
- 285 millilitres mid-strength beer
  (3.5 per cent alcohol content)
- 80 millilitres or 1 *small* glass table wine
  (12 per cent alcohol content)
- 25 millilitres spirits (40 per cent alcohol content)
- 55 millilitres fortified wine such as port.

8   Plant sterols

Plant sterols are naturally occurring compounds that appear in small amounts in fruit, vegetables, legumes, nuts, seeds and oils. As they have a similar structure to cholesterol, if you eat enough of them they compete with cholesterol for absorption. The cholesterol (and sterols) eventually pass through the body without being absorbed, lowering your levels of LDL (bad) cholesterol.

For maximum effect on your blood cholesterol levels you need to eat 2–3 grams of plant sterols each day. On average, this can produce a 10 per cent reduction in your LDL cholesterol levels. Eating more than 3 grams of plant sterols a day will have no further effect on your cholesterol levels. Eating such amounts of plant sterols would be impossible if we had to rely only on conventional foods. Fortunately, a number of plant-sterol-enriched products are now available.

Plant-sterol-enriched foods

Recent advances in 'functional' foods have led to the development of sterol-enriched products. CSIRO has conducted extensive research on these foods. Plant-sterol-enriched margarines, yoghurts and milks are now available. Each serve provides 0.8 grams of plant sterols, so with 3 serves a day of a combination of these products you will reach the 2 gram target easily.

sterol product	1 serve (0.8 grams sterol)
Flora pro-activ Original	10 grams (2 teaspoons)
Flora pro-activ Light	10 grams (2 teaspoons)
Flora pro-activ Ultra Light	10 grams (2 teaspoons)
Flora pro-activ Olive	10 grams (2 teaspoons)
Logicol Regular	10 grams (2 teaspoons)
Logicol Extra Light	10 grams (2 teaspoons)
Logicol Plus Vitamins	10 grams (2 teaspoons)
Nuttelex Pulse	10 grams (2 teaspoons)
Logicol low-fat yoghurt	200 grams
Yoplait Heart Active yoghurt	200 grams
Pura Heart Active milk	250 millilitres

Plant-sterol-enriched foods and CLIP

The CLIP eating plan has been designed to include 3 units of plant-sterol-enriched products each day. This includes 200 grams yoghurt, 250 millilitres milk and 10 grams (2 teaspoons) margarine, which provides 2.4 grams plant sterols each day. If you wish to maximise weight loss, choose light margarine varieties to reduce your energy intake but maintain your sterol intake. See page 116 for some suggested combinations of sterol-enriched foods.

9   Lean protein foods

Protein foods are an essential part of a healthy diet. They are necessary for maintaining our muscles, especially as we get older but also if we are on a weight-loss program. One concern about high-protein diets has been that foods high in protein and fat and low in carbohydrate could harm the heart. Recent research reassures us that eating a lot of protein doesn't damage the heart. In fact, eating more protein foods while limiting our intake of refined carbohydrate foods may be beneficial.

All protein foods also help control hunger, so it is important to eat lean protein foods at each meal. The best protein foods are lean animal sources, such as red meat, chicken and fish, and vegetable sources, such as soy protein. Soy protein was once thought to lower cholesterol levels substantially, but recent studies indicate that eating 50 grams of soy a day lowers LDL cholesterol only by about 3 per cent.

10 Oils and seeds

Some fats, such as the fat in nuts, can be good for you. Oils from some plant sources, such as olive, sunflower, soy, linseed, cottonseed, canola and avocado, can all help lower cholesterol. They are best used to replace fats such as butter, lard, cream, copha and coconut fat, which are all high in saturated fat and increase cholesterol levels.

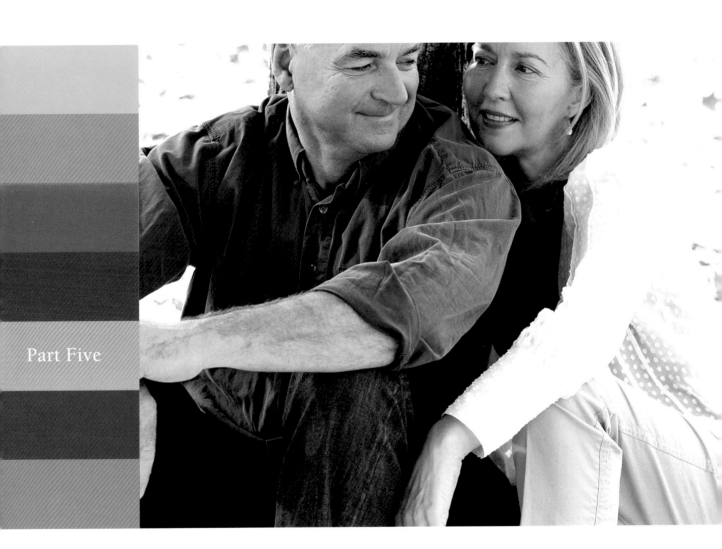

Part Five

CLIP and you

by Xenia Cleanthous, Gemma Williams
and Dr Manny Noakes

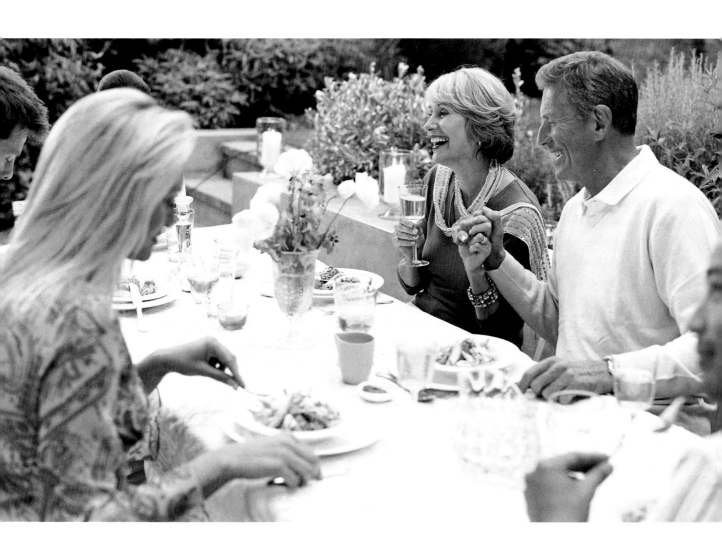

What is the CLIP eating plan?

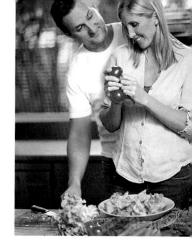

The CLIP eating plan is not just for people who need to lose weight. It is suitable for anyone who wants to reduce their cholesterol and prevent CVD.

CLIP is also great for anyone who wishes to live a healthy lifestyle, whether or not they have high cholesterol. One of the eating plan's key features is that it offers two options for your evening meal. Option 1 is higher in protein, and Option 2 has less protein but also includes carbohydrates. The option you choose is up to you. If you prefer more protein foods, such as lean red meat, chicken and fish, then Option 1 will suit you better. If you would rather have a bit of pasta or rice with your evening meal, then Option 2 is for you. But you don't need to have the same option each night. This provides plenty of variety and flexibility while keeping you healthy. The menu plans on pages 124–49 feature a mixture of both options and the recipes include dinners for both options.

We recognise that some people need more energy from their diet than others, even when they are trying to lose weight and/or lower their cholesterol. For this reason, we have developed four different energy levels within the CLIP eating plan. For more information on these kilojoule levels and on how to determine which you should use, see page 108.

Option 1 or 2 for dinner?

The CLIP eating plan provides two eating styles for the evening meal, both of which are low in saturated fat. These options are set out on page 106. You are free to alternate between the two options or to always eat one or the other.

Option 1 is a high-protein choice that does not include a carbohydrate food with dinner. This option offers a protein allowance of 150 grams lean red meat, chicken, pork, fish, tofu or legumes.

Option 2 offers a combination of 100 grams lean red meat, chicken, pork, fish, tofu or legumes and 80 grams (½ cup) of cooked pasta, rice, potato, noodles or legumes.

You will notice that legumes (baked beans, lentils, kidney beans, and so on) can be eaten either as a protein or a carbohydrate food. We encourage you to include legumes at least twice a week.

If you have high triglyceride levels you may like to choose Option 1 more often, as research has shown that reducing carbohydrate intake can lower blood triglyceride levels.

The CLIP eating plan

The daily requirements and allowances on the CLIP eating plan are summarised on pages 106–107. For the first few weeks we suggest you try to stick as closely as possible to the daily CLIP menu plans (see page 124). This will give you a chance to familiarise yourself with the key features of the CLIP eating plan, and to get into a good routine. Once you feel confident with CLIP, there's more than enough flexibility for you to start getting creative.

It is important to remember that the eating plan has been designed so that each food group provides different key nutrients and benefits. By having each food in the type and amount specified you can be sure you'll be getting a nutritionally complete diet.

Watch your salt intake

Another key feature of the CLIP eating plan is that it is low in salt. Remember to use herbs, lemon and lime juice, vinegar, garlic, pepper and chilli rather than adding salt. Whenever possible, choose salt-reduced varieties of sauces (such as soy, tomato and chilli sauce), stocks and tinned vegetables, and select fish tinned in spring water rather than brine.

CLIP's key foods

The ten super foods you have already read about form the core of the CLIP eating plan and will help you achieve your health and weight-loss goals.

Plant-sterol-enriched foods for extra cholesterol control

Milk, yoghurt and margarine spreads are available at the moment as plant-sterol-enriched products, but new products may become available in the future. The spreads combine healthy polyunsaturated fats with plant sterols to lower cholesterol. Sterol-enriched low-fat milk and yoghurt provide variety, so that you can always be sure to keep your sterol intake at a beneficial level.

If your cholesterol levels are high, the CLIP basic plan can provide 2.4 grams of plant sterols each day, in the form of 3 serves of plant-sterol-enriched products. The simplest way to meet this intake is to consume 250 millilitres (1 serve) sterol-enriched milk, 200 grams (1 serve) sterol-enriched yoghurt and 10 grams (1 serve) sterol-enriched margarine each day. If this seems too daunting, or you don't eat yoghurt for example, there are plenty of other combinations that will help you reach the minimum 2 grams of sterols each day. As long as your 3 serves fit in with the CLIP eating plan, it's up to you which combination you choose. See page 116 for a few suggestions to get you started.

Choose reduced-fat versions of sterol margarines for spreading and melting if you are aiming for maximum weight loss.

The cost of plant-sterol-enriched products is generally higher than that of conventional spreads and dairy foods. If this is an issue for you, you can still gain significant health benefits by choosing non-sterol-enriched margarines rather than butter, and low-fat dairy foods rather than full-fat versions.

Recording your daily intake

Our volunteers have found that a critical component in successful weight loss was recording their daily food intake. We have made this process as painless as possible by providing a simple daily checklist; download it from our website (www.csiro.au/clip) or photocopy Appendix 3 (see page 262). You may like to copy or print it with the basic plan on one side and the checklist on the other, so that you can refer to the diet plan whenever you need to.

Be sure to be as accurate as possible with your checklist. If you eat extra amounts of any foods, you need to write them down. Careful recording assists you in pinpointing where any extra kilojoules might be creeping in.

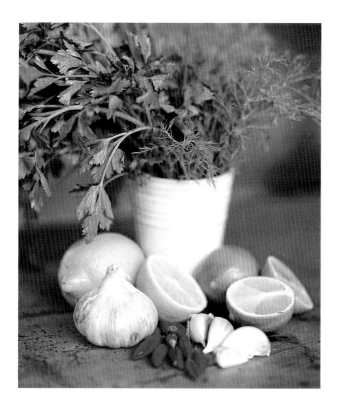

The Free List: anytime foods and drinks

These foods contain minimal kilojoules, so eat them freely to spice up your meals.

Vegetables – all vegetables are free *except* for potato and sweet potato, which need to be treated as part of your dinner carbohydrate allowance.
Drinks – cocoa (made with water), coffee, tea, herbal tea, diet cordial, diet soft drinks, unflavoured mineral water, water.
Condiments – artificial sweeteners, salt-reduced curry powder, diet jelly, diet topping, fat-free salad dressing or mayonnaise, garlic, ginger, herbs, horseradish, lemon, mint sauce, mustard, parsley, low-salt pickles, spices, stock (low-salt only), verjuice, vinegar, wasabi.

Note: A small amount of cornflour, custard powder or sugar is fine for thickening or sweetening dishes. 1 level teaspoon of cornflour, custard or sugar contains 40–60 kilojoules. This is low enough not to worry about if you use them only occasionally. If nuts are used in a recipe in small amounts, it is okay to consider the kilojoule contribution as negligible. Alternatively, you could treat them as part of your nut allowance and consume slightly fewer nuts that day as snacks.

Your daily food allowance on the CLIP basic plan

1 LEAN PROTEIN FOODS FOR DINNER

Either Option 1 = 1½ units a day *or*
Option 2 = 1 unit a day

1 unit is equal to:

• 100 grams any raw lean meat,
  including fish* and chicken

• 100 grams tofu

• 100 grams TVP (see page 112)

• 100 grams cooked legumes

• 2 eggs

* We recommend oily fish for dinner at least twice a week

2 CARBOHYDRATE FOODS FOR DINNER

Either Option 1 = 0 units a day *or*
Option 2 = 1 unit a day

1 unit is equal to:

• 80 grams (½ cup) cooked rice, pasta,
  noodles or couscous (30 grams raw weight)

• 100 grams cooked legumes*

• 1 medium–large potato (150 grams)

• 1 × 40 gram slice wholegrain bread

• 1 slice wholewheat Mountain Bread

• 1 large slice fruit loaf

• crisp bread – 3 × Ryvita *or* 4 × Vita-Weat

* We recommend cooked legumes for dinner at least twice
  a week (counted either as protein or carbohydrate unit)

3 LEAN PROTEIN FOODS FOR LUNCH

½ unit a day

Eat 40 grams (cooked weight; 50 grams raw weight)
of any lean protein source (tinned or fresh fish or
seafood,* chicken, turkey, pork, salt-reduced ham,
beef, lamb or 1 egg) each day for lunch.

* We recommend oily fish for lunch at least twice a week

4 CARBOHYDRATE FOODS FOR LUNCH

2 units a day

1 unit is equal to 1 × 40 gram slice wholegrain bread.

5 HIGH-SOLUBLE-FIBRE CEREAL

1 unit a day

1 unit is equal to 40 grams oats- or psyllium-based
cereal, unsweetened muesli or rolled oats.

6 LOW-FAT DAIRY

2 units a day

1 unit is equal to:

• 250 millilitres (1 cup) low-fat milk*

• 200 grams (1 tub) low-fat or yoghurt*

• 200 grams (1 tub) low-fat custard or low-fat
  dairy dessert

- 250 millilitres (1 cup) soy milk or 200 grams (1 tub) soy yoghurt
- 40 grams (2 slices) reduced-fat (less than 10 per cent fat) cheese

PLUS 2 units cheese a week

1 unit is equal to:
- 20 grams (1 slice) full-fat cheese
- 40 grams (2 slices) reduced-fat cheese

* For extra cholesterol-lowering effect, choose sterol-enriched milk and yoghurt

7   VEGETABLES
At least 2½ units a day from the Free List (see page 105)

1 unit is equal to 1 cup cooked vegetables. We recommend ½ unit salad and 2 units cooked vegetables each day. Aim to include orange and green vegies, such as carrots, pumpkin, spinach and broccoli, to boost your intake of beta-carotenes.

8   FRUIT
2 units a day

1 unit is equal to:
- 150 grams fresh or tinned, unsweetened fruit
- 150 millilitres unsweetened fruit juice
- 30 grams dried fruit

9   NUTS
1 unit a day

1 unit is equal to 20 grams dry-roasted unsalted nuts (2 tablespoons or 15 nuts).

10   FATS AND OILS
5 units a day

1 unit is equal to:
- 1 teaspoon any liquid oil such as canola, olive or sunflower oil.
- 1 teaspoon polyunsaturated or monounsaturated margarine*
- 2 teaspoons light margarine*

3 units can be exchanged for an extra 20 grams nuts or 60 grams avocado

* For extra cholesterol-lowering effect, choose sterol-enriched margarine

11   INDULGENCE FOODS
4 units a week

1 unit is equal to any food or drink providing approximately 450 kilojoules, such as 150 millilitres wine or 20 grams chocolate. See page 264 for more ideas.

If you don't need to lose weight, you can be more liberal with carbohydrate foods, fruit, nuts and oils.

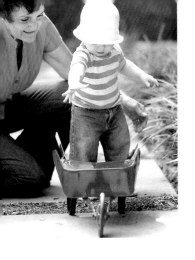

Choosing your kilojoule level for CLIP

Because we all have different kilojoule needs, we have developed different 'levels' of the CLIP eating plan.

Apart from the basic plan on pages 106–107 (level 1 – 5800 kilojoules), there are three other levels, offering 6600, 7600 and 8600 kilojoules respectively. As a general rule, level 1 or 2 will be suitable for most women and level 3 or 4 for most men. There are three basic steps for following the CLIP eating plan.

1 **Determine your kilojoule needs**
   See page 19 for working out your daily kilojoule needs. If you wish to lose weight, make sure you subtract approximately 2000 kilojoules from this figure to lose about 0.5 kilograms a week, or subtract approximately 4000 kilojoules to lose about 1 kilogram a week.

2 **Follow the appropriate level**
   Once you have determined your daily kilojoule needs, choose the level that offers the number of kilojoules nearest to your daily needs. Although the table opposite gives amounts for combining Options 1 and 2, you can choose all Option 1 or all Option 2 without significantly altering the kilojoule count.

3 **Modify the plan to maintain weight**
   See page 120 for the CLIP maintenance plan and tips on how to maintain your new low weight.

If you are uncomfortably hungry and are losing weight too rapidly, try moving up a level. If you feel you are losing weight too slowly and that you would be satisfied with less food, consider dropping down a level.

High cholesterol, normal weight?

Most people think that only overweight people can have high cholesterol, but this is not necessarily the case. If you are within your healthy weight range but still need to lower your cholesterol, fill up on more of the CLIP key foods. These heart-protective foods include nuts and seeds, oils and plant-sterol-enriched margarines, fish, avocado, fruit, vegetables, wholegrain breads, cereals and oats, low-fat dairy products and lean protein foods. Here are a few different approaches you could take.

1 You might like to calculate your daily energy needs (see page 19) so you can choose which of the energy levels best suits your needs.
2 You could follow the maintenance program on page 120. This involves following level 1 of the eating plan and adding extra energy from top-ten foods in 500-kilojoule blocks.
3 You could eat according to hunger, always choosing from the heart-protective foods listed on page 264.

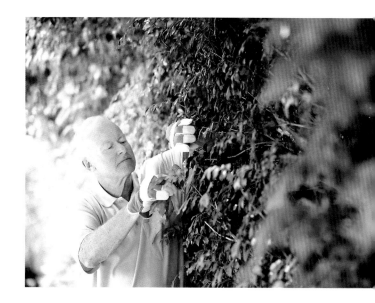

CLIP with Option 2 dinners

level	1	2	3	4
daily energy intake (kilojoules)	5800	6600	7600	8600
protein for dinner (units/day)*	1	1½	1½	1½
carbohydrate for dinner*	1	1	1	1
protein for lunch (units a day)	½	½	½	½
wholegrain bread (units a day)	2	2	2	3
high-soluble-fibre cereal (units a day)	1	1	1½	1½
low-fat dairy (units a day)	2	3	3	3
cheese (units a **week**)	2	2	2	2
vegetables (units a day)	2	2	2	2
salad (units a day)	½	½	½	½
fruit (units a day)	2	3	3	3
fats and oils (units a day)	5	5	5	5
nuts (units a day)	1	1	2	3
indulgences (units a **week**)	4	4	4	4

*CLIP with Option 1 dinners

protein for dinner (units a day)	1½	2	2	2
carbohydrates for dinner (units a day)	0	0	0	0

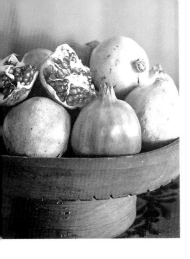

Vegetarians and CLIP

Vegetarian diets are generally low in animal products and high in fruit and vegetables.

The greater amount of plant sources in vegetarian diets also makes them high in dietary fibre and rich in antioxidants and phytonutrients. Research has consistently shown that vegetarians generally have a lower risk of CVD. This seems to arise from a high intake of fruit and vegetables and possibly of shorter-chain plant omega-3 fatty acids, as well as from a healthier lifestyle.

If you are a vegetarian, it is important to ensure that your diet is balanced and contains all the essential nutrients for your optimal health. Here are five important nutrients that vegetarians need to be aware of.

1 Protein

Protein plays many important roles in our bodies, especially in keeping our muscles strong and building up our immune system to protect us from disease. If you eat fish and other seafood, eggs or low-fat dairy, these are all good protein sources. If you are a vegan, you will need to rely on plant protein sources, including legumes, nuts and seeds, whole grains and soy products.

Soy and your heart

You may have heard that the protein in soy products can help lower your cholesterol, but the effect is rather small. The fat from soybeans may, however, help lower cholesterol, and it also contains shorter-chain omega-3 fatty acids. Although soy products may not directly lower your cholesterol, they are still a great source of protein and other nutrients for all diets, vegetarian or not.

2 Iron

Iron helps our red blood cells carry oxygen to our tissues and organs so it can be used to produce energy. Not having enough iron can leave you feeling weak and tired. As iron is mainly found in animal foods such as lean red meat, poultry and fish, some vegetarians become iron-deficient. If you don't eat fish or seafood, it is important to eat a variety of iron-containing plant foods to ensure you are getting sufficient iron. These include legumes, green leafy vegetables, dried fruit, nuts and seeds, wholemeal and wholegrain breads, and iron-enriched cereals. If you eat eggs, the yolk is a source of iron.

3 Calcium

Calcium is essential for keeping your bones and teeth strong and healthy. Too little calcium in the diet can increase the risk of bone fractures and conditions such as osteoporosis. Vegetarians can find calcium in low-fat dairy foods or calcium-enriched soy alternatives, tofu, nuts and seeds (especially almonds and sesame seeds), and some green vegetables, such as broccoli and spinach. If you eat fish, the best options are those with small edible bones, such as tinned salmon and sardines.

4 Zinc

Zinc is a vital mineral for growth and development, particularly for developing a strong immune system. Like iron, zinc is found mainly in animal meats, so some vegetarians can become zinc-deficient. If you eat fish, seafood, low-fat dairy or eggs, these are all good sources of zinc. Good plant sources include legumes, nuts, seeds and whole grains.

5 Vitamin B12

Vitamin B12 is one of the eight members of the B-vitamin complex. It is central to the formation of red blood cells and to normal functioning of the brain and nervous system. Since this vitamin is found naturally only in animal sources, vegans need to supplement their diet with alternative sources, such as B12-enriched cereals and soy products, and/or take Vitamin B12 supplements.

Do you need supplements?

A well-balanced vegetarian diet should provide enough of all the essential nutrients without the need for dietary supplements. This may be more difficult to achieve if you are a vegan. If you are unable to consume enough plant sources of iron, calcium and vitamin B12 (including enriched products), you may need to take supplements for these nutrients. We suggest you consult your doctor to ensure your diet is nutritionally adequate before taking any dietary supplements.

Omega-3s for vegetarians

We know that the right amount of long-chain omega-3 fatty acids (LC omega-3s) from fish and fish oils can help decrease the risk of CVD and other conditions. If you eat fish and seafood, you can of course obtain sufficient amounts of LC omega-3s, especially from oily fish such as sardines, Atlantic salmon, Spanish mackerel and fresh tuna. A vegetarian who does not eat fish or seafood, therefore obtaining only shorter-chain (SC) plant omega-3s from their diet, will find it a little more difficult to gain the benefits that come from LC omega-3s. Our bodies can convert SC omega-3s into the long-chain types found in fish, but this process is not very efficient.

A vegetarian who does not eat fish or seafood can obtain some LC omega-3s from eggs and small amounts of SC omega-3s from canola oil and canola-based margarine spreads, soybean oil, linseed and linseed oil, and walnuts and walnut oil. Although the Heart Foundation suggests at least 2 grams of plant SC omega-3s a day to help reduce the risk of CVD, this intake is recommended in conjunction with 500 milligrams LC omega-3s from fish, seafood or fish oil supplements. If you don't eat fish, you should check the level of LC omega-3s in omega-3-enriched foods such as eggs, bread and dairy products.

In Australia, development of a vegetarian source of LC omega-3s is ongoing, so keep an eye out for new products in your supermarket, pharmacy or health-food shop. Foods containing SC omega-3s are still a great source of polyunsaturated fats and other nutrients, so don't get too hung up about which omega-3s you are eating.

Plant sterols for vegetarians

The Heart Foundation recommends a daily intake of 2–3 grams of plant sterols a day to help lower your cholesterol. If you eat dairy products, you can meet this target by eating sterol-enriched dairy products such as the Pura Heart Active range and the sterol-enriched margarines, such as Logicol or Flora pro-activ. These margarines are not suitable for vegan diets because they contain milk solids. Nuttelex Pulse, however, is a plant-sterol-enriched table spread that does not contain any animal products and is therefore suitable for vegans.

CLIP for vegetarians

The CLIP eating plan is easily modified to incorporate vegetarian options, and the recipes in this book include vegetarian alternatives for lunch and options 1 and 2 for dinner. See page 149 for a sample vegetarian CLIP menu plan. For the protein component of the eating plan, vegetarians should use the following conversions – 100 grams lean meat, poultry or fish is equal to:

- 2 eggs
- 100 grams tofu

- 130 grams prepared textured vegetable protein (TVP) mince, or
- 130 grams cooked legumes

Textured vegetable protein (TVP)

TVP is a meat substitute derived from soybeans. It has a mince-like texture and provides a good low-fat source of protein for vegetarians. It is very versatile and can be used in a variety of dishes, including soups and stews, lasagne, tacos and patties.

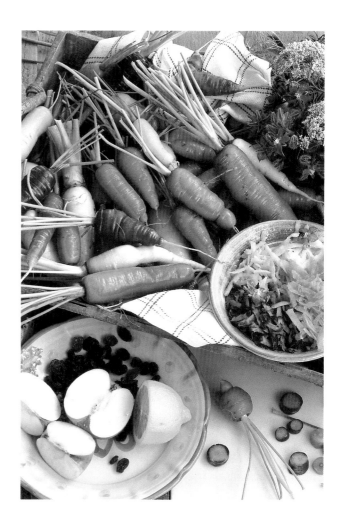

Eating out on CLIP

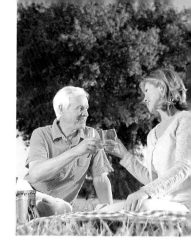

Eating out is an enjoyable and often unavoidable part of life, and there is no reason to stop while you are on the CLIP eating plan.

Try to limit your meals out to once a week if you are following CLIP to lose weight. Once you reach your target weight, the maintenance plan (see page 120) allows more meals out. Here are some simple tips for eating out without ruining all your hard work.

- If your job regularly involves eating out at restaurants for lunch, switch your lunch and evening meals. That way you can stay sociable while still keeping to the eating plan, and it makes for a nice, simple dinner of a sandwich or salad in the evening. If the rest of the family is still eating a regular meal, have some too, but make sure you work out just how many units of carbohydrate and protein you have left for that meal and be extra careful with your portions.
- Take it easy with the alcohol. Alcohol contains plenty of extra kilojoules, so keep within the recommendations. Since our first drink is usually to quench our thirst, start with water. Alternate your alcoholic drinks with mineral water or diet soft drink, and don't allow top-ups – they make

it too difficult to keep track of how much you're drinking. Some people find choosing an extra-tasty (and expensive) glass of wine to savour and enjoy helps slow down their alcohol consumption.

- Practise judging quantities of protein and carbohydrate so that when you are out you are able to estimate how much of the chicken breast you have ordered is equal to 150 grams (Option 1) or 100 grams (Option 2) and leave the excess portion on your plate. Some people find they have to work at changing their mindset to allow them to leave uneaten food on their plate, but the waste is more detrimental in you than in the bin.
- You might like to ask for extra salad or steamed vegetables rather than chips or mash. And don't forget to ask the waiter for no dressings or sauces. Or at least ask for the dressing 'on the side' and make sure you don't add too much.
- Request no bread and butter and remember to count your skim-milk cappuccinos and lattes as dairy units.

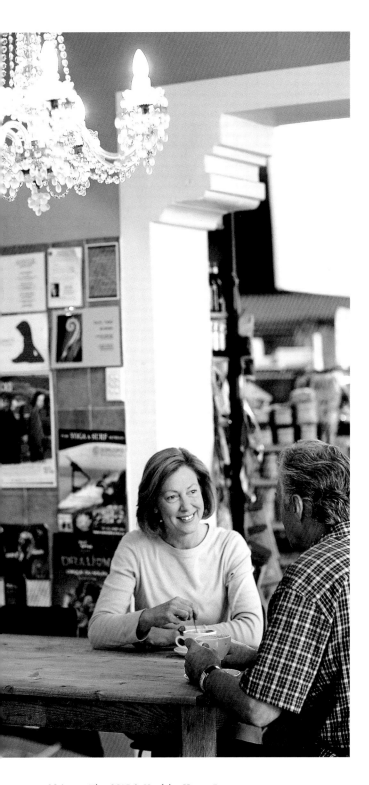

- Choose a fish dish (not battered or fried of course).
- Watch your salt intake – avoid dishes you know will be naturally salty or have lots of salt added.
- If you're having more than one course, choose a vegetable-based soup or salad for your entrée. You could also have two entrées rather than an entrée and a main.
- If you can't resist something sweet, share it with someone else.
- If you are eating at a friend's house, offer to bring the nibbles so you can cater for your own needs. Choose raw or lightly steamed vegetables such as carrots, celery, cucumber, snow peas, mushrooms, cauliflower and broccoli for dipping instead of biscuits. Dips such as carrot and coriander, hummus, tzatziki, beetroot and eggplant can be lower in kilojoules than other more traditional, cream-cheese-based dips. Try the dip recipes in the recipe section of this book.
- Don't let yourself get over-hungry before you go to a cocktail or dinner party. Before you start to nibble, take a look at what's on offer and decide which you will eat and which to avoid. Position yourself away from the food at parties. Slow down your eating and concentrate on the conversations.

The CLIP eating plan: frequently asked questions

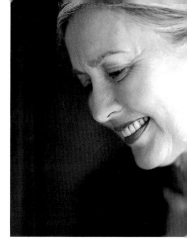

How long before I see a reduction in my cholesterol?

Studies have shown that changing your diet can lower your cholesterol in as little as 2 weeks. Nevertheless, it is important to remember that your responsiveness depends on many factors, such as your initial cholesterol levels, your weight and your activity level.

Can my cholesterol level get too low?

No. Small amounts of cholesterol are needed by your body but your liver makes enough to meet these needs independent of what you eat.

Is the CLIP eating plan suitable for everyone?

The CLIP eating plan is aimed primarily at adults with a high cholesterol level. It may not be suitable for people with special nutritional needs, such as babies, children and pregnant or nursing mothers. If you are concerned, consult your doctor to check whether the eating plan is suitable for you.

Is CLIP suitable if I want to lose weight but don't have high cholesterol?

The CLIP eating plan is suitable for anyone who wants to lose weight by following a healthy eating plan. You can still include the sterol-enriched products, but standard margarines and low-fat dairy products would also be fine.

Which dinner option is best if I have high triglyceride levels?

Research suggests that if you have elevated triglyceride levels you could benefit from a lower-carbohydrate diet. If your triglyceride levels are high, choose the higher-protein, lower-carbohydrate dinner option (Option 1).

I like variety. Can I alternate the dinner options?

Certainly. You do not have to stay with the same dinner option for any set period of time and it is up to you which dinner option you choose. You may like to go with the same one each evening or to change depending on the day.

Can I change the order of the meals and the foods eaten?

Of course. Some components of the eating plan can be quite tricky to start with, so you might like to begin by keeping to the basic structure of each main meal. But once you are confident about the eating plan, feel free to get those creative juices flowing. As long as you eat all the specified foods (see pages 106–107), you do not have to eat them in any set order, but a regular eating routine will make it easier to stick to the eating plan. The most important thing is to keep to the units and portions outlined in the plan. You may prefer to combine your snacks with your main meals or to swap lunch with dinner.

Can I use the Total Wellbeing Diet recipes for the CLIP eating plan?

Certainly. Books 1 and 2 both provide excellent recipes that would need only minor adjustments to be suitable for the CLIP eating plan. They will be particularly useful if you choose Option 1 at dinner, but remember to adjust the recipe to suit serving and portion sizes.

Will the plant sterols still work if I do not have the full portions of the required foods?

Yes, but not as effectively as the full portions. To maximise their impact on your cholesterol, we recommend consuming 2 grams of plant sterols each day. The CLIP eating plan provides 2.4 grams of plant sterols each day.

Which sterol margarine should I choose?

Sterol margarines are currently available in 'original' and light varieties. The light varieties have less total fat and saturated fat, which also means they have fewer kilojoules. There is no difference in their sterol content; each variety provides 0.8 grams of plant sterol per 10 grams of margarine. If you aim to lose weight, the light varieties would be more suitable. For the original sterol margarines, 1 unit = 1 teaspoon (5 grams), and for the light varieties, 1 unit = 2 teaspoons (10 grams).

Which oil is best?

A variety of oils are suitable for the CLIP eating plan. Choose oils that are low in saturated fat and higher in monounsaturated and polyunsaturated fats, such as olive, canola, sunflower, safflower, soybean and corn oils. You can also use oils derived from nuts and seeds, such as almond, peanut, macadamia, walnut, grapeseed and sesame oils. Each has a unique flavour.

How can I meet the dairy requirements?

Low-fat dairy foods are excellent sources of protein and calcium. You can reach your daily dairy target (2–3 units) simply by having low-fat milk on your cereal and a tub of low-fat yoghurt for afternoon tea. You could also use low-fat milk to make custard and sauces. Try low-fat custards and diet dairy desserts, fromage frais and calcium-enriched soy alternatives. Indulge in a skim-milk latte or hot chocolate. Low-fat flavoured milks (sugar-free) would also be suitable. You could make white sauce or curry with fat-free evaporated milk.

Are all lean meats suitable for lunch protein?

Nearly. Deli-sliced varieties, such as roast beef, chicken, turkey and pork are all suitable, as long as they are trimmed of fat. You should generally limit your intake of ham and corned beef (silverside) because of their high salt content. You can also eat tinned fish, including tuna, salmon and sardines, but ensure they are tinned in spring water rather than brine; 98 per cent fat-free flavoured varieties would also be suitable. You could also eat fish tinned in oil instead of using salad dressing or margarine on your sandwich and count it as part of your fat and oil units for the day.

Legumes appear in the protein *and* the carbohydrate section. Why is this?

Legumes are a unique food – not only are they packed with essential vitamins and minerals, but they are also an excellent plant source of protein *and* carbohydrates. Try to incorporate legumes into your meal plan at least twice a week. 1 unit protein = 100 grams cooked legumes; 1 unit carbohydrate = 100 grams cooked legumes.

How can I include my nut portion?

You don't have to rely only on eating dry-roasted nuts to obtain your nut units. There are many nut spreads and pastes on the market that are suitable. Supermarkets and health-food shops sell nut and seed pastes such as peanut butter, almond paste, cashew paste and tahini (sesame seed paste), but choose low-salt varieties. You can also use seeds such as pumpkin, linseed, sesame and sunflower seeds for your nut unit. Sprinkle them on your cereal, yoghurt and salads, or add them to stir-fries. Dry-roasted varieties are also suitable for snacks. 1 unit nuts = 20 grams nuts, seeds, or 3 teaspoons nut paste or spread.

I have heard that linseed is good for your heart. Can this be included on the diet?

Yes. Linseed is an excellent source of short-chain omega-3 fatty acids and fibre, especially soluble fibre. Look out for it as an ingredient in breads and cereals. You can also buy it on its own or in a ground mix of linseed, sunflower seeds and almonds (LSA). You can use linseed or LSA mix as part of your daily 1 unit nuts (20 grams = 20 grams nuts). Sprinkle it on cereal, salads or even your vegies, or mix it into yoghurt.

Are some fruit or vegetables better than others?

Research has consistently shown that a high intake of fruit and vegetables can protect against CVD. To maximise your intake of essential vitamins, minerals, antioxidants and other vital components of vegetables, it is best to eat a variety of different-coloured fruit and generous serves of vegetables each day. As a rule of thumb, aim to eat two fruits and five vegetables each day. Red, orange and yellow fruits and vegetables tend to be high in carotenoids, which our bodies use to make vitamin A. Dark green leafy vegetables are generally high in folic acid, one of the nutrients that keeps our DNA healthy. Always include a liberal amount of vegetables with your meals, in salads or soups, or lightly steamed or stir-fried.

Isn't cheese high in saturated fat? Why is it included in the CLIP eating plan?

Cheese is an excellent source of protein and calcium and, as it contains minimal lactose, it is a great dairy option for people who are lactose intolerant. Most cheeses are high in saturated fat, salt and kilojoules, so it is important to control how much and what type of cheese you eat. This is why we have limited full-fat cheese to twice a week. There are many lower-fat varieties, however, that would be suitable for the CLIP eating plan on a daily basis. Always read the nutrition panel to make sure the cheese contains less than 10 grams of fat per 100 grams (that is, less than 10 per cent fat). 1 unit cheese = 20 grams full-fat or 40 grams reduced-fat or low-fat cheese.

Can I eat eggs if I have high cholesterol?

Sure. Even though eggs contain dietary cholesterol, research shows that this has little impact on the cholesterol levels in most people's blood. Eggs are a great

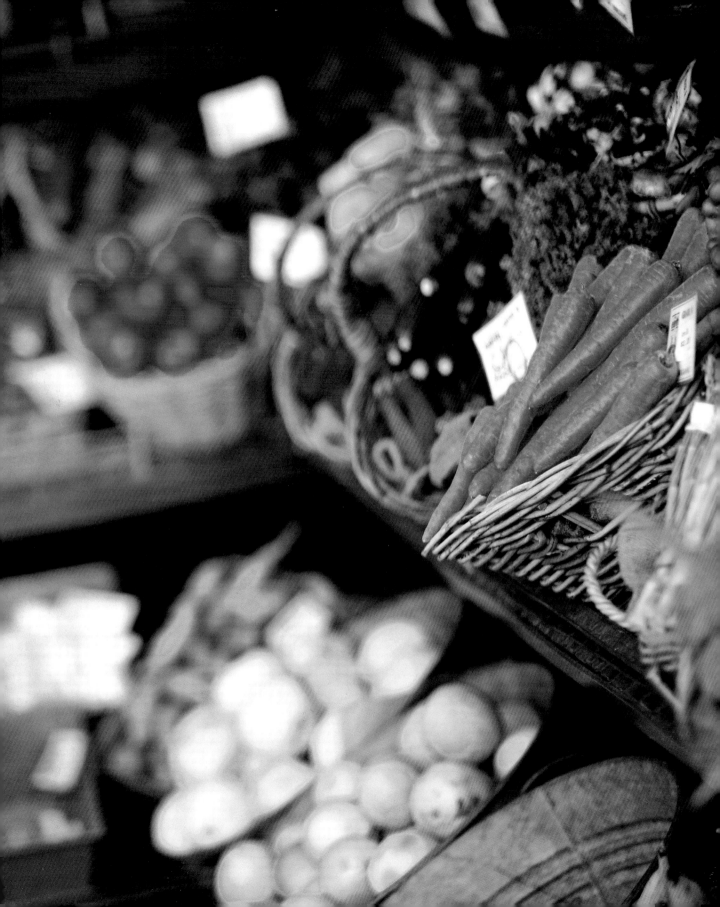

low-saturated-fat source of good-quality protein and other nutrients such as vitamin A, the B-group vitamins, LC omega-3s and the antioxidants lutein and zeaxanthin. They are easy to store and cook, and are very affordable. You can eat up to 6 eggs a week while on CLIP. You could have them in a sandwich at lunchtime or make a vegetable frittata (see page 154) for dinner. 1 egg = ½ unit protein.

What are the benefits of omega-3-enriched eggs?

Omega-3-enriched eggs are produced by hens that have been fed a diet of polyunsaturated fats and kelp. It's worth checking the nutrition panel for the fat content of these eggs, but they are certainly a good way to boost your omega-3 intake. If you are a vegetarian you should bear in mind that the oils fed to the chickens come from fish and seafood sources.

Can tea really protect my heart?

Tea contains a group of antioxidant compounds called polyphenols, which can lower the risk of CVD by reducing the damage caused by LDL cholesterol. Black and green teas are particularly high in several antioxidant compounds. One group of these antioxidants, flavonols, are also found in some fruits and vegetables, and wine. A high dietary intake of flavonols may be associated with a reduced risk of death from CVD. We have no conclusive answers, however, as to how tea specifically may be protective. Studies indicate that a slightly decreased risk occurs in people who drink three or more cups a day.

Is chocolate actually good for you?

Possibly yes, but only in moderation. Dark chocolate contains high amounts of cocoa, which is rich in polyphenols. These substances have been associated with reduced blood pressure in some studies. But even dark chocolate is high in saturated fat. High-saturated-fat foods can increase your cholesterol, but half the saturated fat in high-cocoa dark chocolate is of a type called stearic acid, which appears to have little effect on blood cholesterol. Despite this, it is still important to remember that the sugar and fat makes it a high-energy food. Drinking hot cocoa made with skim milk will give you the benefits of cocoa without the extra kilojoules of chocolate. If you are on the CLIP eating plan, however, you can eat chocolate as an indulgence unit (25 grams dark chocolate = 1 unit indulgence; 4 units indulgence allowed each week on the basic plan).

Which is better, margarine or butter?

Margarine is high in healthy unsaturated fats, which makes it a much better choice than butter or some dairy blends, which are high in saturated fat. You may have heard that the manufacturing process for margarine produces trans fatty acids, a type of fat thought to increase LDL cholesterol. The good news is that these have been phased out in Australian margarines. Check the nutrition panel before you buy, and look for margarines low in saturated fat that contain less than 1 per cent trans fatty acids. If the product has the Heart Foundation Tick, it's a good choice.

Is it 'margarine' or 'margarine spread'?

Fewer spreads are simply labelled 'margarine' these days. This is because margarine is defined as containing at least 80 per cent fat, and since many spreads now contain less than this they must be referred to as 'margarine spread'. The best options for lowering your cholesterol are the sterol-enriched varieties. Try the reduced-fat versions of these to maximise weight loss.

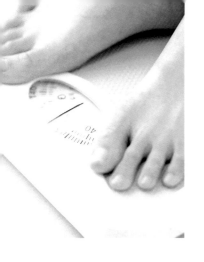

The CLIP weight and cholesterol maintenance plan

Once you have reached your target weight, the real challenge begins – to keep the weight off and your cholesterol down forever.

Ensure that you have regular check-ups with your doctor to monitor your CVD risk factors. You may need to take cholesterol-lowering medication (see page 26) in the long term, despite having reached a healthier weight, but don't feel disheartened. The CLIP maintenance plan will complement your medication nicely for ongoing control of your cholesterol levels, blood pressure and weight.

We have found that the most effective way to maintain a new weight after following a weight-loss program is to add new foods to the basic eating plan slowly. We all have different energy needs, so there will be a period of trial and error until you work out how much you can eat to maintain your new weight. We suggest slowly adding new foods to your daily menus in 500-kilojoule 'blocks' of heart-protective foods (see the table on page 264 for ideas).

The CLIP weight and cholesterol maintenance plan gives you the flexibility to maintain the core eating plan in the long term, freeing you from worry that your weight and cholesterol will creep up again.

Adding 500-kilojoule blocks on the maintenance plan

Here's how you should go about gradually incorporating 500-kilojoule blocks into your eating plan over a 3-week period and beyond.

week 1	Add 1 × 500-kilojoule block to your basic daily plan. This means that each day you eat 500 kilojoules more than you did before.
week 2	If you're still losing weight, add another 500-kilojoule block to your daily food allowance.
week 3	If you're still losing weight (lucky you!), add another 500-kilojoule block to your daily allowance and continue doing this each week until you maintain your weight.

If you start to gain weight again, do not add any foods the following week. If your weight gain is more than 1 kilogram, drop back to the previous week's plan. Once you reach a stage where your weight is stable, that should remain your eating plan for long-term weight maintenance. You will need to weigh yourself weekly during this phase to judge properly the effect of adding extra foods to your eating plan. Once you have achieved a stable weight, however, it's best to avoid obsessing over the scales – weighing yourself once a fortnight is more than enough.

And keep exercising. This will be the key to maintaining your healthy weight and managing your CVD risk factors forever.

5 weeks on the maintenance plan

Here is one way that extra 500-kilojoule blocks might be added to the CLIP eating plan after weight loss. Of course, if you want to eat a different 500-kilojoule block each day, you can. Just make sure you keep using the maintenance plan daily checklist in Appendix 4 (see page 263 or download from www.csiro.au/clip) to keep track of your food intake until you've worked out your maintenance requirements. Continue adding blocks only if you are still losing weight. As soon as your weight stabilises, stop adding blocks.

week 1 maintenance	choose any 1 block, e.g. a large slice of toast at breakfast
week 2 maintenance	if still losing weight, choose any 2 blocks, e.g. large slice of toast + a piece of fruit as a snack
week 3 maintenance	if still losing weight, choose any 3 blocks, e.g. large slice of toast, fruit + extra nuts/seeds
week 4 maintenance	if still losing weight, choose any 3 blocks + 1 indulgence unit, e.g. large slice of toast, fruit, nuts/seeds + 25 grams dark chocolate
week 5 maintenance	if still losing weight, choose any 3 blocks + 2 indulgence units, e.g. large slice of toast, fruit, nuts/seeds, dark chocolate + 150 millilitre glass of wine

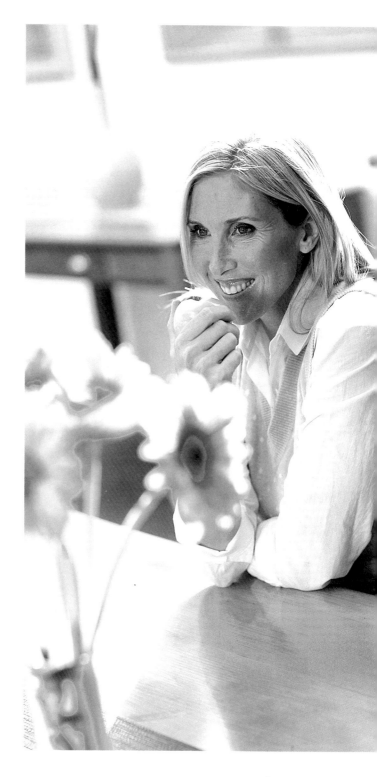

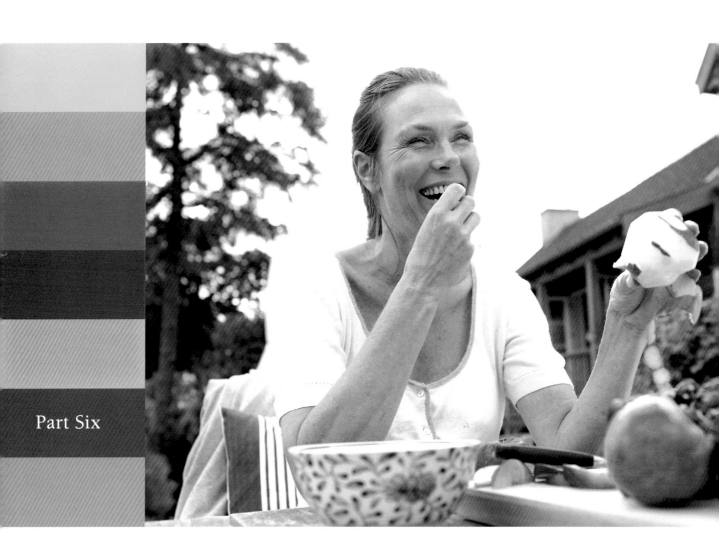

Part Six

CLIP menu plans

by Xenia Cleanthous and Gemma Williams

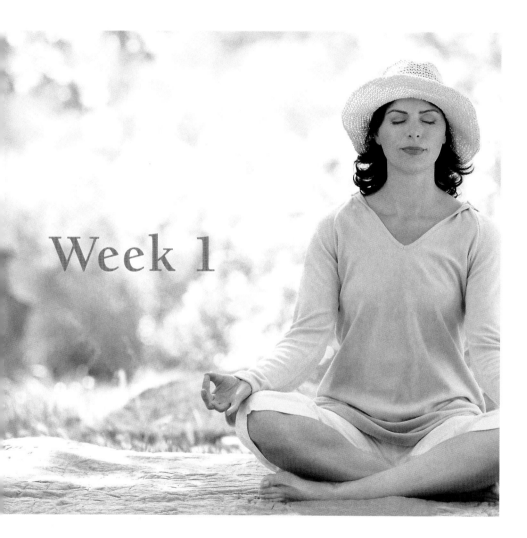

Week 1

DAILY SNACK

Choose from these snack options each day. You *must* eat the 2 units fruit and the 1 unit dairy each day to ensure your daily food allowance is complete. Always add the 1 unit nuts even if nuts are included in the menu plan for that day.

- tea or coffee with low-fat milk
- 200 g low-fat yoghurt (1 unit dairy)
- 300 g fresh fruit (2 units fruit)
- 20 g dry-roasted, unsalted nuts (1 unit nuts)

Week 1	Breakfast	Lunch	Dinner
Monday	40 g high-soluble-fibre cereal (e.g. Kellogg's Guardian) with 250 ml low-fat sterol milk	Roast beef & salad sandwich (2 slices wholegrain bread with 2 tsp sterol spread, 40 g shaved roast beef, low-salt pickles & ½ cup salad leaves)	150 g fish: Fish & Vegetable Skewers (see p 179) 1 cup green salad with 40 g avocado & fat-free dressing
Tuesday	40 g unsweetened untoasted muesli with 250 ml low-fat sterol milk	Pizza with Tomato, Artichoke & Mushrooms (see p 163)	150 g lamb: Winter Lamb Casserole (see p 194) 1½ cups steamed pumpkin greens with 2 tsp sterol spread
Wednesday	40 g instant oats with 250 ml low-fat sterol milk	Smoked Trout Salad with Orange, Green Beans & Horseradish (see p 158) 1 extra slice wholegrain bread with 2 tsp sterol spread	OPTION 2 – 100 g chicken, 80 g cooked rice: Chicken & Vegetable Paella (see p 220)
Thursday	40 g high-soluble-fibre cereal (e.g. Uncle Tobys Healthwise) with 250 ml low-fat sterol milk	Bean salad (140 g tinned mixed beans with 60 g avocado, 1 cup salad leaves, ½ cup mixed red & green capsicum, sweet corn & fat-free balsamic dressing) Cheese on toast (1 slice wholegrain bread, 2 tsp sterol spread & 20 g cheddar)	OPTION 2 – 100 g beef, 80 g cooked pasta: substitute beef for chicken in Sesame Chicken with Soba Noodles & Plum Sauce (see p 224)
Friday	40 g unsweetened toasted muesli with 250 ml low-fat sterol milk	Smoked trout sandwich (2 slices wholegrain bread with 2 tsp sterol spread, 40 g smoked trout, 20 g avocado, red onion & ½ cup baby cos lettuce)	150 g pork: Stir-fried pork with green beans & mixed mushrooms (see p 190)
Saturday	40 g high-soluble-fibre cereal (e.g. Uncle Tobys Oatbrits) with 20 g nuts & 250 ml low-fat sterol milk	Shaved turkey sandwich (2 slices wholegrain bread with 2 tsp sterol spread, 40 g turkey, 20 g avocado, 1 tsp cranberry sauce, ½ cup baby cos lettuce & sliced tomato)	150 g beef: Barbecued Sirloin with Mustard Crust & Portobello Mushrooms (see p 183) 1½ cups rocket salad with fat-free dressing
Sunday	40 g instant oats with 12 g nuts & 250 ml low-fat sterol milk	Egg & salad sandwich (2 slices wholegrain bread with 2 tsp sterol spread, 1 hard-boiled egg, fat-free mayonnaise, sliced spring onion & ½ cup salad leaves)	OPTION 2 – 100 g fish, 100 g cooked legumes: Chargrilled Salmon with Lentils, Spinach & Yoghurt (see p 211)

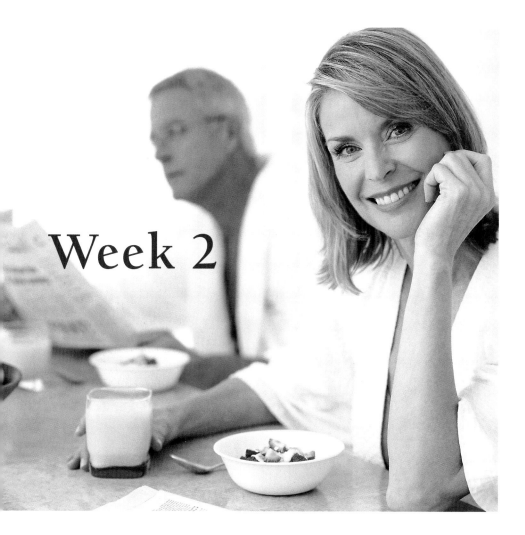

Week 2

DAILY SNACK

Choose from these snack options each day. You *must* eat the 2 units fruit and the 1 unit dairy each day to ensure your daily food allowance is complete. Add the 1 unit nuts even if nuts are included in the menu plan for that day. On Sunday the dinner recipe includes ½ unit fruit, so take this into account when choosing your snacks on that day.

- tea or coffee with low-fat milk
- 200 g low-fat yoghurt (1 unit dairy)
- 300 g fresh fruit (2 units fruit)
- 20 g dry-roasted, unsalted nuts (1 unit nuts)

Week 2	Breakfast	Lunch	Dinner
Monday	40 g unsweetened untoasted muesli with 250 ml low-fat sterol milk	Carrot & Ginger Soup (see p 168) 100 g salt-reduced baked beans on 1 slice wholegrain bread with 2 tsp sterol spread	150 g chicken: Spiced Chicken Casserole (see p 189) 1 cup steamed green beans & broccoli tossed in 1 tsp sesame oil
Tuesday	40 g high-soluble-fibre cereal (e.g. Kellogg's Guardian) with 250 ml low-fat sterol milk	Beef or chicken wrap (1 whole-wheat Mountain Bread wrap with 40 g roast beef or chicken, 1 tbsp low-fat hummus & 1 cup tabouli)	OPTION 2 – 100 g beef, 150 g potato: rub a sirloin steak with 2 tsp oil & herbs, then grill or barbecue 1 baked potato & 1½ cups baked carrot, onion & zucchini with 2 tsp sterol spread melted over
Wednesday	40 g instant oats with 250 ml low-fat sterol milk	Curried egg roll (1 wholegrain roll [80 g] with 2 tsp sterol spread, 1 egg mashed with 2 tsp fat-free mayonnaise, low-salt curry powder, lemon juice & ½ cup salad leaves)	150 g fish: Marinated Fish Skewers with Capsicum & Fennel Salad (see p 183)
Thursday	40 g unsweetened toasted muesli with 250 ml low-fat sterol milk	Zucchini & Pea Fritters with Smoked Salmon & Herbs (see p 163), the fritters shallow-fried in 2 tsp sterol spread	OPTION 2 – 100 g lamb, 100 g cooked legumes: Slow-cooked Lamb Shanks with Beans, Carrots & Spring Onions (see p 228) 1 cup steamed broccoli & green beans drizzled with 2 tsp sesame oil
Friday	40 g high-soluble-fibre cereal (e.g. Uncle Tobys Healthwise) with 250 ml low-fat sterol milk	Ham, cheese & salad sandwich (2 slices wholegrain bread with 2 tsp sterol spread, 40 g salt-reduced ham, 20 g cheddar & ½ cup salad leaves)	150 g fish: Roasted Salmon Salad with Minted Chilli Dressing (see p 186)
Saturday	40 g high-soluble-fibre cereal (e.g. Uncle Tobys Oatbrits) with 20 g nuts & 250 ml low-fat sterol milk	Tuna, ricotta & lettuce sandwich (2 slices wholegrain bread with 2 tsp sterol spread, 40 g tuna tinned in spring water, 40 g low-fat ricotta, ½ cup chopped lettuce & sliced celery & red onion)	OPTION 2 – 100 g chicken, 100 g cooked legumes: Smoked Chicken, Green Bean & Lentil Salad with Sesame Seeds (see p 220)
Sunday	40 g instant oats with 20 g nuts & 250 ml low-fat sterol milk	Chicken, Snow Pea & Pumpkin Salad (see p 164) with 1 tsp sterol spread on the bread	150 g pork: Pork cutlets with Cabbage, Parsnips & Raisins (see p 192)

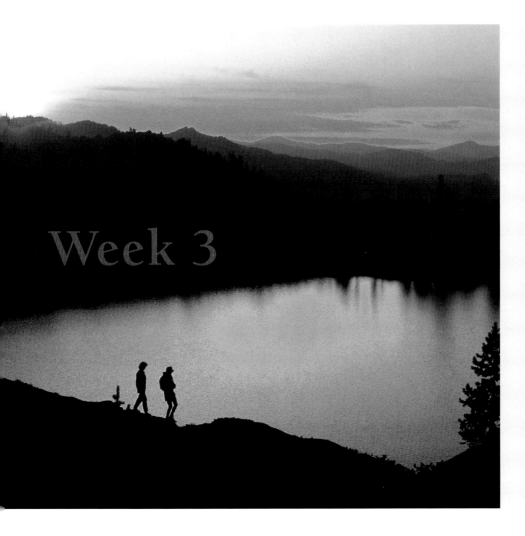

Week 3

DAILY SNACK

Choose from these snack options each day. You *must* eat the 2 units fruit and the 1 unit dairy each day to ensure your daily food allowance is complete. Add the 1 unit nuts even if nuts are included in the menu plan for that day. A unit breakdown is provided for each recipe after the cooking instructions.

- tea or coffee with low-fat milk
- 200 g low-fat yoghurt (1 unit dairy)
- 300 g fresh fruit (2 units fruit)
- 20 g dry-roasted, unsalted nuts (1 unit nuts)

Week 3	Breakfast	Lunch	Dinner
Monday	40 g instant oats with 250 ml low-fat sterol milk	Salmon sandwich (2 slices wholegrain bread with 2 tsp sterol spread, 40 g salmon tinned in spring water, gherkin, lemon juice & ½ cup rocket leaves)	150 g beef: Chargrilled Beef with Zucchini, Pine Nuts & Spinach (see p 178) 1 cup salad vegetables with 3 tsp olive oil & balsamic vinegar
Tuesday	40 g unsweetened untoasted muesli with 250 ml low-fat sterol milk	Chicken pita pockets (1 small wholegrain pita bread [80 g] with 2 tsp sterol spread, 40 g sliced chicken breast, 2 tsp low-fat natural yoghurt, dried or fresh mint, sliced cucumber & tomato & ½ cup lettuce)	OPTION 2 – 100 g lamb, 100 g cooked legumes: rub a lamb steak with 3 tsp oil & herbs, then grill or barbecue 1½ cups salad vegetables with 100 g salt-reduced tinned chickpeas & fat-free dressing
Wednesday	40 g high-soluble-fibre cereal (e.g. Kellogg's Guardian) with 12 g nuts & 250 ml low-fat sterol milk	Beef, cheese & tomato toasted sandwich (2 slices wholegrain bread with 2 tsp sterol spread, 40 g shaved roast beef, 20 g cheddar & sliced tomato)	150 g seafood: Prawn & Tomato Soup with Mussels (see p 180)
Thursday	40 g high-soluble-fibre cereal (e.g. Uncle Tobys Healthwise) with 20 g nuts & 250 ml low-fat sterol milk	Egg salad with croutons (1 slice wholegrain bread spread with 1 tsp sterol spread then toasted & chopped into squares, 1 chopped hard-boiled egg, 2 tsp fat-free mayonnaise, 1½ cups chopped lettuce, celery & red onion) 2 wholegrain crisp bread with 1 tsp sterol spread	OPTION 2 – 100 g fish, 150 g potato: Baked Snapper Fillets with Lemon & Thyme Potatoes (see p 213)
Friday	40 g unsweetened toasted muesli with 250 ml low-fat sterol milk	Roasted Carrot, Tofu & Fennel Salad (see p 160) 2 wholegrain crisp bread with 2 tsp sterol spread	OPTION 2 – 100 g chicken, 80 g cooked noodles: Sesame Chicken with Soba Noodles & Plum Sauce (see p 224)
Saturday	40 g instant oats with 250 ml low-fat sterol milk	Hot & Sour Pumpkin Soup (see p 168) with toasted ham, cheese & tomato sandwich (2 slices wholegrain bread with 2 tsp sterol spread, 40 g salt-reduced ham, 20 g cheddar & sliced tomato)	150 g beef: rub a sirloin steak with 3 tsp oil & herbs, then grill or barbecue 1½ cups baked mixed vegetables
Sunday	**BRUNCH** Sweet Corn & Potato Rösti with Smoked Trout & Roasted Tomatoes (see p 155) 4 wholegrain crisp bread with 2 tsp sterol spread 1 low-fat latte or low-fat cappuccino		150 g lamb: Oregano & Lemon Lamb with Green Beans & Butternut Pumpkin (see p 194)

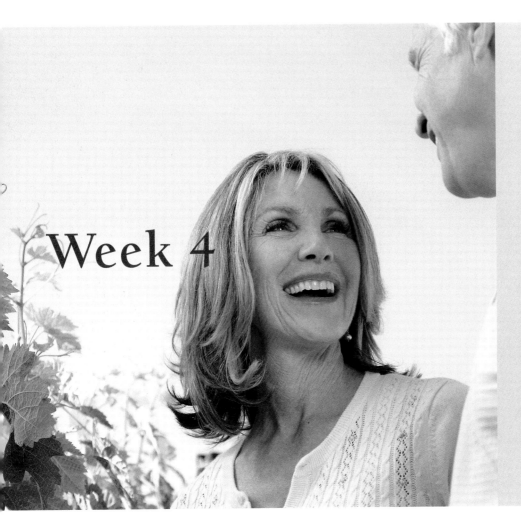

Week 4

DAILY SNACK

Choose from these snack options each day. You *must* eat the 2 units fruit and the 1 unit dairy each day to ensure your daily food allowance is complete. Add the 1 unit nuts even if nuts are included in the menu plan for that day. On Tuesday the dinner includes ½ unit fruit and on Wednesday the dinner includes 1 unit fruit.

- tea or coffee with low-fat milk
- 200 g low-fat yoghurt (1 unit dairy)
- 300 g fresh fruit (1 unit fruit)
- 20 g dry-roasted, unsalted nuts (1 unit nuts)

On Friday, the dinner recipe includes ½ unit indulgence.

Week 4	Breakfast	Lunch	Dinner
Monday	40 g high-soluble-fibre cereal (e.g. Uncle Tobys Oatbrits) with 250 ml low-fat sterol milk	Tuna & bean salad (40 g tuna tinned in spring water, 100 g tinned beans, 1 cup mixed salad vegetables, 2 tsp fat-free mayonnaise) 2 wholegrain crisp bread with 2 tsp sterol spread	150 g chicken: Sticky Chicken Drumsticks (see p 184) 1½ cups mixed vegetables stir-fried in 2 tsp olive oil
Tuesday	40 g high-soluble-fibre cereal (e.g. Kellogg's Guardian) with 250 ml low-fat sterol milk	Mixed salad with cheese (½ cup chopped tomato & cucumber with ½ cup lettuce, 20 g low-salt feta & fat-free dressing) Baked beans on toast (1 slice wholegrain bread, 2 tsp sterol spread & 140 g salt-reduced baked beans)	150 g pork: Braised Pork with Dried Cherries (see p 190) 1½ cups steamed mixed vegetables tossed in 1 tsp sesame oil
Wednesday	40 g unsweetened toasted muesli with 250 ml low-fat sterol milk	Beef or chicken & salad sandwich (2 slices wholegrain bread with 2 tsp sterol spread, 40 g roast beef or chicken, 20 g avocado & ½ cup salad leaves)	150 g fish: Hot Smoked Salmon, Watercress & Pink Grapefruit Salad (see p 184)
Thursday	40 g instant oats with 20 g nuts & 250 ml low-fat sterol milk	Pork & salad roll (1 wholegrain roll [80 g] with 2 tsp sterol spread, 40 g shaved roast pork, 2 tsp apple sauce, sliced tomato & red onion & ½ cup salad leaves)	OPTION 2 – 100 g chicken, 80 g cooked rice: Smoked Chicken, Green Bean & Lentil Salad with Sesame Seeds (see p 220) with an extra 1 tsp sesame seeds and 1 tsp olive oil added with the dressing
Friday	40 g unsweetened untoasted muesli with 250 ml low-fat sterol milk	Sardine sandwich (2 slices wholegrain bread with 2 tsp sterol spread, 40 g sardines tinned in spring water, 20 g avocado & 1 cup red capsicum, red onion & tomato)	OPTION 2 – 100 g beef, 150 g potato: Beef & Guinness Casserole (see p 232)
Saturday	40 g instant oats with 250 ml low-fat sterol milk	Turkey roll (1 wholegrain roll [80 g] with 2 tsp sterol spread, 40 g shaved turkey, 20 g Swiss cheese, 1 tsp cranberry sauce, ½ cup lettuce & sliced cucumber)	OPTION 2 – 100 g lamb, 150 g potato: rub a lamb steak with 3 tsp oil & herbs, then grill or barbecue 1 baked sweet potato (150 g) 1½ cups baked carrots, onion & zucchini
Sunday	40 g high-soluble-fibre cereal (e.g. Uncle Tobys Healthwise) with 250 ml low-fat sterol milk	Egg & salad sandwich (2 slices wholegrain bread with 2 tsp sterol spread, 1 hard-boiled egg, 20 g avocado, sliced spring onion & ½ cup salad leaves)	150 g seafood: Chargrilled Squid Salad (see p 179)

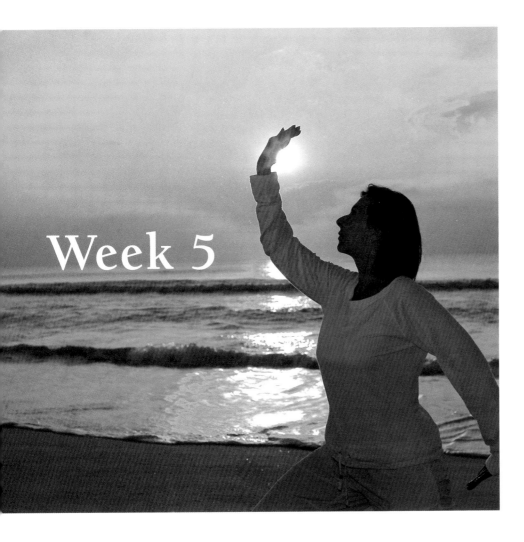

Week 5

DAILY SNACK

Choose from these snack options each day. You *must* eat the 2 units fruit and the 1 unit dairy each day to ensure your daily food allowance is complete. Note that dinner on Friday includes ½ unit dairy, so take this into account when choosing your snacks for Friday. Add the 1 unit nuts even if nuts are included in the menu plan for that day.

- tea or coffee with low-fat milk
- 200 g low-fat yoghurt (1 unit dairy)
- 300 g fresh fruit (2 units fruit)
- 20 g dry-roasted, unsalted nuts (1 unit nuts)

Week 5	Breakfast	Lunch	Dinner
Monday	40 g instant oats with 5 g nuts & 250 ml low-fat sterol milk	Curried egg sandwich (2 slices wholegrain bread with 2 tsp sterol spread, curried egg – 1 egg mashed with 2 tsp fat-free mayonnaise, low-salt curry powder & lemon juice – ½ cup watercress & sliced cucumber)	150 g fish: Roasted Gemfish with Saffron & Cardamom Pumpkin (see p 186)
Tuesday	40 g high-soluble-fibre cereal (e.g. Uncle Tobys Oatbrits) with 20 g nuts & 250 ml low-fat sterol milk	Smoked chicken & bean salad (40 g shaved smoked chicken, 100 g tinned beans, 1½ cups mixed salad vegetables & fat-free dressing) 2 wholegrain crisp bread with 2 tsp sterol spread	OPTION 2 – 100 g beef, 80 g cooked pasta: substitute beef for chicken in Sesame Chicken with Soba Noodles & Plum Sauce (see p 224)
Wednesday	40 g high-soluble-fibre cereal (e.g. Kellogg's Guardian) with 250 ml low-fat sterol milk	Salmon salad (40 g salmon tinned in spring water, 40 g low-fat ricotta, sweet corn, chopped tomato & green beans & ½ cup salad leaves with fat-free salad dressing) 1 wholegrain bread roll (80 g) with 2 tsp sterol spread	OPTION 2 – 100 g pork, 80 g cooked rice: Indian Pork Curry with Minted Yoghurt & Basmati Rice (see p 228)
Thursday	40 g high-soluble-fibre cereal (e.g. Uncle Tobys Healthwise) with 250 ml low-fat sterol milk	Carrot & Ginger Soup (see p 168) with toasted beef, cheese & tomato sandwich (2 slices wholegrain bread with 2 tsp sterol spread, 40 g shaved roast beef, 20 g cheddar & sliced tomato)	150 g lamb: Chargrilled Lamb Fillets with Pepperonata (see p 197) 1 cup steamed mixed vegetables drizzled with 1 tsp sesame oil
Friday	40 g unsweetened toasted muesli with 250 ml low-fat sterol milk	Bruschetta with Hummus, Roasted Vegetables & Basil (see p 160)	OPTION 2 – 100 g fish, 150 g potato: Fish Chowder (see p 213) 1½ cups green salad tossed in 1 tsp sesame oil
Saturday	40 g instant oats with 250 ml low-fat sterol milk	Pork & coleslaw sandwich (2 slices wholegrain bread with 2 tsp sterol spread, 40 g shaved roast pork, ½ cup coleslaw with 2 tsp fat-free mayonnaise)	150 g beef: Thai Beef Kebabs (see p 192) 1 cup Sesame Spinach Salad (see p 199) using 3 tsp sesame oil
Sunday	40 g unsweetened untoasted muesli with 5 g nuts & 250 ml low-fat sterol milk	Tuna sandwich (2 slices wholegrain bread with 2 tsp sterol spread, 40 g tuna tinned in spring water, 2 tsp fat-free mayonnaise, sliced celery & spring onions & ½ cup lettuce)	150 g chicken: Sumac-roasted Chicken with Beetroot & Almond Salad (see p 189)

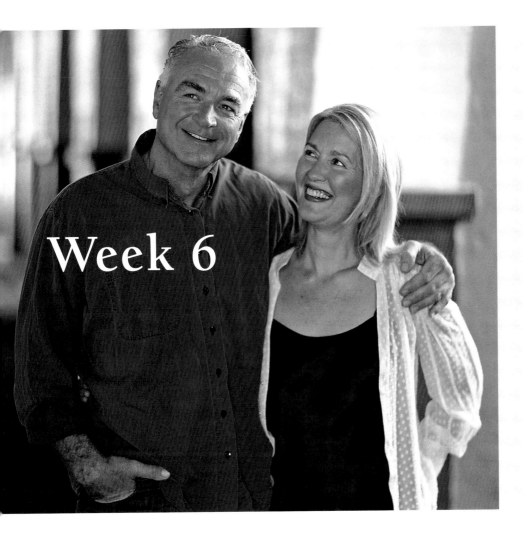

Week 6

DAILY SNACK

Choose from these snack options each day. You *must* eat the 2 units fruit and the 1 unit dairy each day to ensure your daily food allowance is complete.

- tea or coffee with low-fat milk
- 200 g low-fat yoghurt (1 unit dairy)
- 300 g fresh fruit (2 units fruit)
- 20 g dry-roasted, unsalted nuts (1 unit nuts)

Week 6	Breakfast	Lunch	Dinner
Monday	40 g high-soluble-fibre cereal (e.g. Uncle Tobys Oatbrits) with 250 ml low-fat sterol milk	Roast chicken roll (1 wholegrain roll [80 g] with 2 tsp sterol spread, 40 g roast chicken, sliced red capsicum & tomato & ½ cup salad leaves)	OPTION 2 – 100 g tuna, 80 g cooked rice: Tuna, Corn & Coriander Patties (see p 224) 1½ cups green salad drizzled with 2 tsp olive oil & a little balsamic vinegar
Tuesday	40 g instant oats with 250 ml low-fat sterol milk	Turkey sandwich (2 slices wholegrain bread with 2 tsp sterol spread, 40 g shaved turkey, alfalfa sprouts, sliced tomato, 60 g avocado & ½ cup rocket leaves)	150 g lamb: Lamb & Spinach Meatballs with Spicy Tomato Sauce (see p 197) 1½ cups mixed salad vegetables
Wednesday	40 g unsweetened untoasted muesli with 250 ml low-fat sterol milk	Smoked trout sandwich (2 slices wholegrain bread with 2 tsp sterol spread, 40 g smoked trout, 40 g avocado, red onion & ½ cup baby cos lettuce)	OPTION 2 – 100 g beef, 40 g bread: Chargrilled Steak Sandwiches with Tomato Relish (see p 232) 1 cup green salad with fat-free dressing
Thursday	40 g instant oats with 250 ml low-fat sterol milk	Vegie Burger with Herb Aïoli (see p 158), the patty shallow-fried in 2 tsp sterol spread	150 g pork: Stir-fried Pork with Green Beans & Mixed Mushrooms (see p 190)
Friday	40 g unsweetened toasted muesli with 250 ml low-fat sterol milk	Ham & cheese toasted sandwich (2 slices wholegrain bread with 2 tsp sterol spread, 40 g salt-reduced ham, 20 g cheddar & sliced tomato & gherkin) ½ cup mixed salad vegetables with fat-free dressing	150 g beef: rub a sirloin steak with 3 tsp oil & herbs, then grill or barbecue 1 cup mixed salad vegetables with fat-free dressing
Saturday	40 g high-soluble-fibre cereal (e.g. Uncle Tobys Healthwise) with 250 ml low-fat sterol milk	Tuna salad (40 g tuna tinned in spring water, sliced cucumber & gherkin, 1 cup salad leaves & 2 tsp fat-free mayonnaise) 4 wholegrain crisp bread with 2 tsp sterol spread	OPTION 2 – 100 g chicken, 80 g burghul: Harissa Chicken with Tabouli (see p 223)
Sunday	BRUNCH Pea, Leek & Mint Frittata (see p 154) 2 wholegrain crisp bread with 1 tsp sterol spread 1 low-fat latte or low-fat cappuccino		150 g seafood: Prawn & Cucumber Salad with Mango (see p 180)

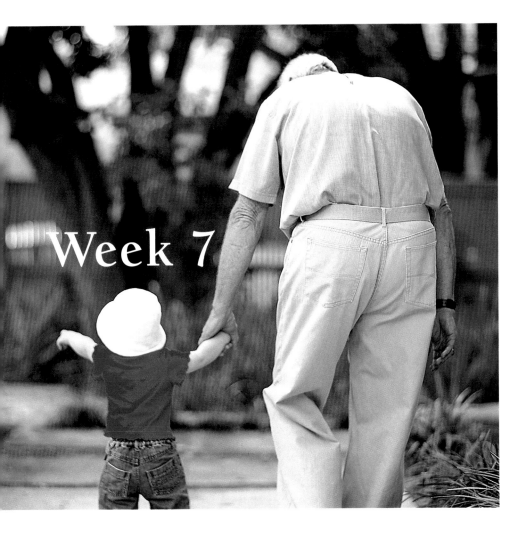

Week 7

DAILY SNACK

Choose from these snack options each day. You *must* eat the 2 units fruit and the 1 unit dairy each day to ensure your daily food allowance is complete. The dinner recipe on Monday includes ½ unit dairy, so take this into account when choosing snacks. Add the 1 unit nuts even if nuts are included for that day.

- tea or coffee with low-fat milk
- 200 g low-fat yoghurt (1 unit dairy)
- 300 g fresh fruit (1 unit fruit)
- 20 g dry-roasted, unsalted nuts (1 unit nuts)

Note that on Wednesday the dinner recipe includes ½ unit indulgence.

40 g high-soluble-fibre cereal (e.g. Kellogg's Guardian) with 250 ml low-fat sterol milk	Roast beef & salad sandwich (2 slices wholegrain bread with 2 tsp sterol spread, 40 g shaved roast beef, low-salt pickles & ½ cup mixed salad vegetables)	OPTION 2 – 100 g fish, 80 g cooked pasta: Tuna Pasta Bake (see p 215) 1½ cups green salad drizzled with 1 tsp olive oil & a little balsamic vinegar
40 g unsweetened untoasted muesli with 12 g nuts & 250 ml low-fat sterol milk	Turkey sandwich (2 slices wholegrain bread with 2 tsp sterol spread, 40 g turkey, 20 g avocado, 1 tsp cranberry sauce, ½ cup baby cos lettuce & sliced tomato)	OPTION 2 – 100 g chicken, 80 g noodles: Sesame Chicken with Soba Noodles & Plum Sauce (see p 224)
40 g unsweetened toasted muesli with 250 ml low-fat sterol milk	Smoked trout sandwich (2 slices wholegrain bread with 2 tsp sterol spread, 40 g smoked trout, 20 g avocado, ½ cup baby cos lettuce & sliced tomato)	OPTION 2 – 100 g beef, 150 g potato: Beef & Guinness Casserole (see p 232)
40 g instant oats with 250 ml low-fat sterol milk	Pizza with Tomato, Artichoke & Mushrooms (see p 163)	150 g lamb: rub a lamb steak with 3 tsp oil & herbs, then grill or barbecue 1½ cups steamed mixed vegetables with 2 tsp sterol spread
40 g high-soluble-fibre cereal (e.g. Uncle Tobys Healthwise) with 5 g nuts & 250 ml low-fat sterol milk	Scrambled egg & baked beans on toast (1 slice wholegrain bread with 1 tsp sterol spread, 1 scrambled egg cooked in 1 tsp sterol spread, 100 g salt-reduced baked beans, grilled tomato & mushrooms)	150 g fish: Roasted Gemfish with Saffron & Cardamom Pumpkin (see p 186)
40 g high-soluble-fibre cereal (e.g. Uncle Tobys Oatbrits) with 250 ml low-fat sterol milk	Pork & salad roll (1 wholegrain roll [80 g] with 2 tsp sterol spread, 40 g shaved roast pork, 60 g avocado, sliced tomato & red onion & ½ cup salad leaves)	OPTION 2 – 100 g chicken, 80 g cooked rice: Smoked Chicken, Green Bean & Lentil Salad with Sesame Seeds (see p 220)
40 g instant oats with 250 ml low-fat sterol milk	Smoked Trout Salad with Orange, Green Beans & Horseradish (see p 158) 2 wholegrain crisp bread with 2 tsp sterol spread	150 g lamb: Lamb & Spinach Meatballs with Spicy Tomato Sauce (see p 197) 1½ cups white bean salad (mixed salad vegetables, 100 g white beans & fat-free dressing)

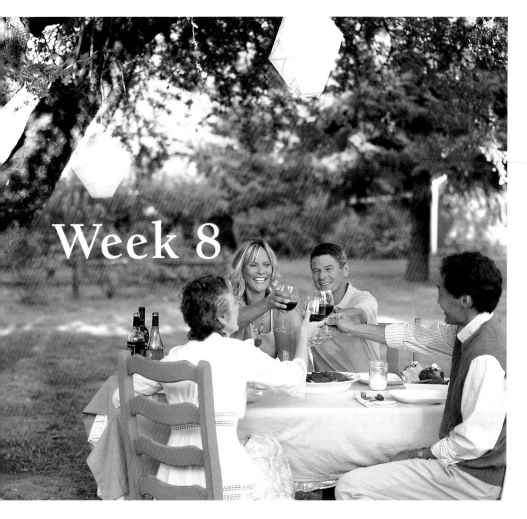

Week 8

DAILY SNACK

Choose from these snack options each day. You *must* eat the 2 units fruit and the 1 unit dairy each day to ensure your daily food allowance is complete. Add the 1 unit nuts even if nuts are already included in the menu plan for that day.

- tea or coffee with low-fat milk
- 200 g low-fat yoghurt (1 unit dairy)
- 300 g fresh fruit (2 units fruit)
- 20 g dry-roasted, unsalted nuts (1 unit nuts)

Week 8	Breakfast	Lunch	Dinner
Monday	40 g unsweetened untoasted muesli with 250 ml low-fat sterol milk	Carrot & Ginger Soup (see p 168) 100 g salt-reduced baked beans on 1 slice wholegrain bread spread with 1 tsp sterol spread	OPTION 2 – 100 g pork, 150 g potato: Fennel & Rosemary Pork with Wilted Spinach & Roast Potatoes (see p 226)
Tuesday	40 g high-soluble-fibre cereal (e.g. Kellogg's Guardian) with 5 g nuts & 250 ml low-fat sterol milk	Roast chicken & cheese roll (1 wholegrain roll [80 g] with 2 tsp sterol spread, 40 g roast chicken, 20 g cheddar, mustard, sliced red capsicum & tomato & ½ cup salad leaves)	150 g seafood: Chargrilled Squid Salad (see p 179)
Wednesday	40 g unsweetened toasted muesli with 250 ml low-fat sterol milk	Egg & salad sandwich (2 slices wholegrain bread with 2 tsp sterol spread, 1 hard-boiled egg, 2 tsp fat-free mayonnaise, sliced spring onion & ½ cup salad leaves)	150 g chicken: Spiced Chicken Casserole (see p 189) 1 cup steamed beans & broccoli tossed in 1 tsp sesame oil
Thursday	40 g instant oats with 250 ml low-fat sterol milk	Zucchini & Pea Fritters with Smoked Salmon & Herbs (see p 163)	150 g beef: rub a sirloin steak with 3 tsp oil & herbs then grill or barbecue 1½ cups steamed vegetables with 2 tsp sterol spread melted over
Friday	40 g high-soluble-fibre cereal (e.g. Uncle Tobys Healthwise) with 250 ml low-fat sterol milk	Chicken, Snow Pea & Pumpkin Salad (see p 164)	OPTION 2 – 100 g seafood, 80 g cooked rice: Prawn & Salmon Risotto with Lemon & Zucchini (see p 218) with 2 tsp sterol spread stirred in at end of cooking
Saturday	40 g instant oats with 250 ml low-fat sterol milk	Ham & salad sandwich (2 slices wholegrain bread with 2 tsp sterol spread, 40 g salt-reduced ham, 20 g cheddar & ½ cup salad leaves)	OPTION 2 – 100 g beef, 40 g bread: rub a sirloin steak with 3 tsp oil & grill or barbecue, then serve on 1 slice toasted wholegrain bread with wholegrain mustard, ½ cup cooked mushrooms, sliced onion 1½ cups mixed salad vegetables
Sunday	40 g high-soluble-fibre cereal (e.g. Uncle Tobys Oatbrits) with 250 ml low-fat sterol milk	Smoked trout sandwich (2 slices wholegrain bread with 2 tsp sterol spread, 40 g smoked trout, 20 g avocado, red onion & ½ cup baby cos lettuce)	150 g lamb: Chargrilled Lamb Fillets with Pepperonata (see p 197) 1 cup steamed mixed vegetables

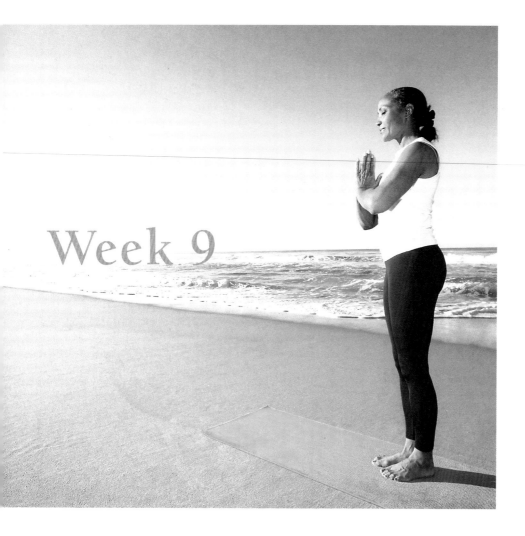

Week 9

DAILY SNACK

Choose from these snack options each day. You *must* eat the 2 units fruit and the 1 unit dairy each day to ensure your daily food allowance is complete. On Thursday the dinner recipe includes ½ fruit unit, so take this into account when choosing your snacks. Add the 1 unit nuts even if nuts are included in the menu plan for that day.

- tea or coffee with low-fat milk
- 200 g low-fat yoghurt (1 unit dairy)
- 300 g fresh fruit (2 units fruit)
- 20 g dry-roasted, unsalted nuts (1 unit nuts)

40 g high-soluble-fibre cereal (e.g. Uncle Tobys Healthwise) with 250 ml low-fat sterol milk	Salmon & bean salad (40 g salmon tinned in spring water, 100 g tinned mixed beans, 20 g avocado, sweet corn, chopped tomato & green beans & ½ cup salad leaves with fat-free salad dressing) 1 slice wholegrain bread with 1 tsp sterol spread	150 g pork: Pork Cutlets with Cabbage, Parsnips & Raisins (see p 192)
40 g instant oats with 12 g nuts & 250 ml low-fat sterol milk	Beef, cheese & tomato toasted sandwich (2 slices wholegrain bread with 2 tsp sterol spread, 40 g shaved roast beef, 20 g cheddar & ½ cup sliced tomato) 1 cup green salad with fat-free dressing	OPTION 2 – 100 g chicken, 100 g legumes: Smoked Chicken, Green Bean & Lentil Salad with Sesame Seeds (see p 220)
40 g unsweetened toasted muesli with 250 ml low-fat sterol milk	Tuna sandwich (2 slices wholegrain bread with 2 tsp sterol spread, 40 g tuna tinned in spring water, 2 tsp fat-free mayonnaise, sliced celery & spring onions & ½ cup butter lettuce)	150 g lamb: Oregano & Lemon Lamb with Green Beans & Butternut Pumpkin (see p 194)
40 g unsweetened untoasted muesli with 250 ml low-fat sterol milk	Roasted Carrot, Tofu & Fennel Salad (see p 160) 2 wholegrain crisp bread with 2 tsp sterol spread	150 g pork : Braised Pork with Dried Cherries (see p 190)
40 g high-soluble-fibre cereal (e.g. Kellogg's Guardian) with 250 ml low-fat sterol milk	Chicken pita pockets (1 small wholegrain pita bread [80 g] with 2 tsp sterol spread, 40 g sliced chicken breast, 2 tsp low-fat natural yoghurt, dried mint, sliced tomato & cucumber & ½ cup lettuce)	OPTION 2 – 100 g fish, 80 g couscous: Dukkah-crusted Salmon with Couscous (see p 216) 1½ cups steamed mixed vegetables drizzled with 3 tsp sesame oil
40 g instant oats with 250 ml low-fat sterol milk	Hot & Sour Pumpkin Soup (see p 168) with toasted ham & tomato sandwich (2 slices wholegrain bread with 2 tsp sterol spread, 40 g salt-reduced ham & sliced tomato)	150 g beef: rub a sirloin steak with 3 tsp oil & herbs, then grill or barbecue 1½ cups baked mixed vegetables
Pea, Leek & Mint Frittata (see p 154) 2 wholegrain crisp bread with 1 tsp sterol spread 20 g nuts 1 low-fat latte or low-fat cappuccino		OPTION 2 – 100 g fish, 150 g potato: Baked Snapper Fillets with Lemon & Thyme Potatoes (see p 213)

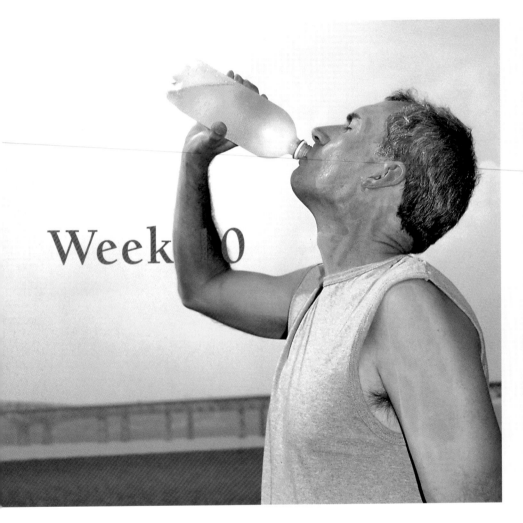

Week 10

DAILY SNACK

Choose from these snack options each day. You *must* eat the 2 units fruit and the 1 unit dairy each day to ensure your daily food allowance is complete. Dinner on Friday includes ½ unit dairy, so take this into account when choosing your dairy snack on that day. Add the 1 unit nuts even if nuts are included in the menu plan.

- tea or coffee with low-fat milk
- 200 g low-fat yoghurt (1 unit dairy)
- 300 g fresh fruit (2 units fruit)
- 20 g dry-roasted, unsalted nuts (1 unit nuts)

Week 10	Breakfast	Lunch	Dinner
Monday	40 g high-soluble-fibre cereal (e.g. Kellogg's Guardian) with 5 g nuts & 250 ml low-fat sterol milk	Roast chicken sandwich (2 slices wholegrain bread with 2 tsp sterol spread, 40 g roast chicken, 20 g cheddar, low-salt pickles & ½ cup salad leaves)	OPTION 2 – 100 g seafood, 150 g potato: Prawn & Salmon Risotto with Lemon & Zucchini (see p 218) 1 cup baked pumpkin
Tuesday	40 g unsweetened toasted muesli with 250 ml low-fat sterol milk	Pork & salad roll (1 wholegrain roll [80 g] with 2 tsp sterol spread, 40 g shaved roast pork, 40 g avocado, sliced tomato & 1 cup salad leaves)	OPTION 2 – 100 g lamb, 100 g legumes: Slow-cooked Lamb Shanks with Beans, Carrots & Spring Onions (see p 228)
Wednesday	40 g instant oats with 250 ml low-fat sterol milk	Sardine sandwich (2 slices wholegrain bread with 2 tsp sterol spread, 40 g sardines tinned in spring water, 1 cup sliced red capsicum, red onion & tomato)	150 g chicken: Sumac-roasted Chicken with Beetroot & Almond Salad (see p 189)
Thursday	40 g unsweetened untoasted muesli with 250 ml low-fat sterol milk	Curried egg roll (1 wholegrain roll [80 g] with 2 tsp sterol spread, 1 egg mashed with 2 tsp fat-free mayonnaise, low-salt curry powder, lemon juice & ½ cup salad leaves)	150 g pork: Stir-fried Pork with Green Beans & Mixed Mushrooms (see p 190)
Friday	40 g high-soluble-fibre cereal (e.g. Uncle Tobys Healthwise) with 20 g nuts & 250 ml low-fat sterol milk	Roast beef sandwich (2 slices wholegrain bread with 2 tsp sterol spread, 40 g lean roast beef, grated fresh horseradish – or salt-reduced prepared horseradish – mixed with 2 tsp fat-free mayonnaise, ½ cup watercress, tomato & grated carrot)	OPTION 2 – 100 g fish, 80 g cooked rice: Thai Green Fish Curry (see p 211)
Saturday	40 g high-soluble-fibre cereal (e.g. Uncle Tobys Oatbrits) with 250 ml low-fat sterol milk	Turkey roll (1 wholegrain roll [80 g] with 2 tsp sterol spread, 40 g shaved turkey, 1 tsp cranberry sauce, sliced cucumber & ½ cup salad leaves)	150 g lamb: coat lamb cutlets in 1 tbsp olive oil & dried rosemary, then grill or barbecue 2 cups steamed mixed vegetables
Sunday	40 g instant oats with 20 g nuts & 250 ml low-fat sterol milk	Tuna & bean salad (40 g tuna tinned in spring water, 100 g tinned beans, ½ cup halved cherry tomatoes, sliced red onion, 1 cup salad leaves, 20 g low-salt feta & fat-free balsamic dressing) 2 wholegrain crisp bread with 2 tsp sterol spread	150 g beef: Barbecued Sirloin with Mustard Crust & Portobello Mushrooms (see p 183) 1 cup rocket salad with fat-free dressing

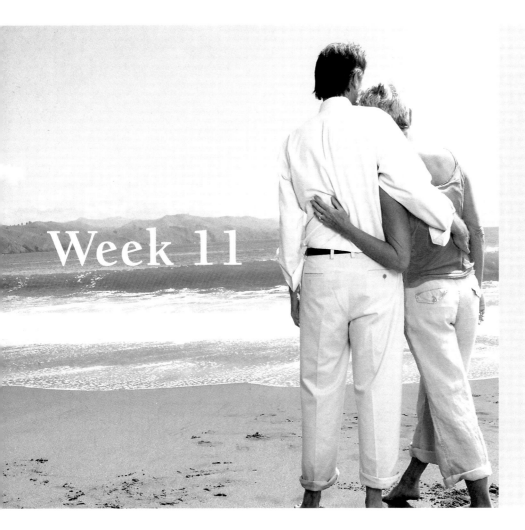

Week 11

DAILY SNACK

Choose from these snack options each day. You *must* eat the 2 units fruit and the 1 unit dairy each day to ensure your daily food allowance is complete. Add the 1 unit nuts even if nuts are included in the menu plan for that day.

- tea or coffee with low-fat milk
- 200 g low-fat yoghurt (1 unit dairy)
- 300 g fresh fruit (2 units fruit)
- 20 g dry-roasted, unsalted nuts (1 unit nuts)

Week 11	Breakfast	Lunch	Dinner
Monday	40 g high-soluble-fibre cereal (e.g. Uncle Tobys Oatbrits) with 250 ml low-fat sterol milk	Salmon sandwich (2 slices wholegrain bread with 2 tsp sterol spread, 40 g salmon tinned in spring water, sliced gherkin & tomato, lemon juice & ½ cup rocket leaves)	150 g lamb: Winter Lamb Casserole (see p 194)
Tuesday	40 g instant oats with 250 ml low-fat sterol milk	Hot & Sour Pumpkin Soup (see p 168) with toasted beef, cheese & tomato sandwich (2 slices wholegrain bread with 2 tsp sterol spread, 40 g shaved roast beef, 20 g cheddar & sliced tomato)	OPTION 2 – 100 g pork, 80 g cooked rice: Indian Pork Curry with Minted Yoghurt & Basmati Rice (see p 228)
Wednesday	40 g unsweetened toasted muesli with 250 ml low-fat sterol milk	Bruschetta with Hummus, Roasted Vegetables & Basil (see p 160)	150 g fish: Roasted Salmon Salad with Minted Chilli Dressing (see p 186), the salmon cooked in 2 tsp sterol spread
Thursday	40 g high-soluble-fibre cereal (e.g. Uncle Tobys Healthwise) with 250 ml low-fat sterol milk	Pork & coleslaw sandwich (2 slices wholegrain bread with 2 tsp sterol spread, 40 g shaved roast pork & ½ cup coleslaw – shredded cabbage & carrot with 2 tsp fat-free mayonnaise)	OPTION 2 – 100 g beef, 40 g bread: Chargrilled Steak Sandwiches with Tomato Relish (see p 232) 1 cup salad leaves drizzled with 2 tsp oil & a little balsamic vinegar
Friday	40 g unsweetened untoasted muesli with 250 ml low-fat sterol milk	Smoked chicken salad (40 g shaved smoked chicken with 40 g avocado, cherry tomatoes, sliced spring onion & celery & fat-free dressing) 4 wholegrain crisp bread with 2 tsp sterol spread	OPTION 2 – 100 g fish, 100 g legumes: Chargrilled Salmon with Lentils, Spinach & Yoghurt (see p 211)
Saturday	40 g instant oats with 20 g nuts & 250 ml low-fat sterol milk	Curried egg sandwich (1 wholegrain bread roll [80 g] with 2 tsp sterol spread, curried egg – 1 egg mashed with 2 tsp fat-free mayonnaise, low-salt curry powder & lemon juice – ½ cup watercress & sliced cucumber)	OPTION 2 – 100 g beef, 80 g cooked pasta: substitute beef for chicken in Sesame Chicken with Soba Noodles & Plum Sauce (see p 224)
Sunday	40 g high-soluble-fibre cereal (e.g. Kellogg's Guardian) with 250 ml low-fat sterol milk	Tuna & bean salad (40 g tuna tinned in spring water, 100 g tinned beans, ½ cup halved cherry tomatoes, sliced red onion, 1 cup salad leaves, 20 g low-salt feta & fat-free balsamic dressing) 2 wholegrain crisp bread with 2 tsp sterol spread	150 g chicken: Sticky Chicken Drumsticks (see p 184) 1½ cups steamed mixed vegetables drizzled with 3 tsp sesame oil

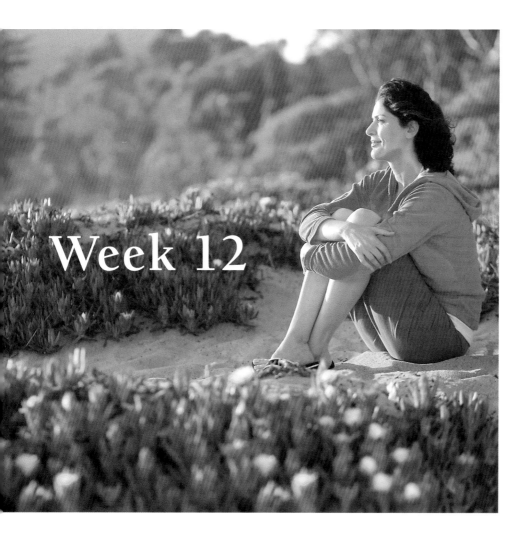

Week 12

DAILY SNACK

Choose from these snack options each day. You *must* eat the 2 units fruit and the 1 unit dairy each day to ensure your daily food allowance is complete. Add the 1 unit nuts even if nuts are included in the menu plan for that day.

- tea or coffee with low-fat milk
- 200 g low-fat yoghurt (1 unit dairy)
- 300 g fresh fruit (2 units fruit)
- 20 g dry-roasted, unsalted nuts (1 unit nuts)

Week 12	Breakfast	Lunch	Dinner
Monday	40 g unsweetened untoasted muesli with 12 g nuts & 250 ml low-fat sterol milk	Salmon salad (40 g salmon tinned in spring water, 20 g ricotta, sweet corn, chopped tomato & green beans & 1 cup salad leaves with fat-free salad dressing) 1 wholegrain roll (80 g) with 2 tsp sterol spread	OPTION 2 – 100 g lamb, 100 g legumes: Thyme & Lemon Lamb Cutlets with Zucchini & Chickpea Salad (see p 230)
Tuesday	40 g instant oats with 250 ml low-fat sterol milk	Ham & cheese toasted sandwich (2 slices wholegrain bread with 2 tsp sterol spread, 40 g salt-reduced ham, 20 g cheddar, sliced tomato & gherkin) ½ cup mixed salad vegetables with 60 g avocado & fat-free dressing	OPTION 2 – 100 g chicken, 80 g cooked rice: Chicken & Vegetable Paella (see p 220)
Wednesday	40 g unsweetened toasted muesli with 250 ml low-fat sterol milk	Egg salad with croutons (1 slice wholegrain bread toasted & chopped into squares, 1 chopped hard-boiled egg, 2 tsp fat-free mayonnaise, 1 cup chopped lettuce, celery & red onion) 2 wholegrain crisp bread with 2 tsp sterol spread	OPTION 2 – 100 g seafood, 80 g cooked pasta: Linguine with Crab, Lime & Coriander (see p 218) 1 cup salad leaves drizzled with 1 tsp olive oil & a little balsamic vinegar
Thursday	40 g high-soluble-fibre cereal (e.g. Uncle Tobys Healthwise) with 250 ml low-fat sterol milk	Beef wrap (1 wholewheat Mountain Bread wrap with 2 tsp sterol spread, 40 g roast beef, 1 cup tabouli & 40 g low-fat hummus)	150 g lamb: substitute lamb for beef in Thai Beef Kebabs (see p 192) 1 cup Sesame Spinach Salad (see p 199) using 2 tsp sesame oil
Friday	40 g instant oats with 250 ml low-fat sterol milk	Vegie Burger with Herb Aïoli (see p 158), the patty cooked in 2 tsp sterol spread	150 g seafood: Prawn & Cucumber Salad with Mango (see p 180)
Saturday	40 g high-soluble-fibre cereal (e.g. Uncle Tobys Oatbrits) with 250 ml low-fat sterol milk	Turkey sandwich (2 slices wholegrain bread with 2 tsp sterol spread, 40 g shaved turkey, alfalfa sprouts, sliced tomato, 40 g avocado & ½ cup rocket leaves)	150 g beef: Chargrilled Beef with Zucchini, Pine Nuts & Spinach (see p 178)
Sunday	**BRUNCH** Sweet Corn & Potato Rösti with Smoked Trout & Roasted Tomatoes (see p 155) 4 wholegrain crisp bread with 2 tsp sterol spread 1 low-fat latte or low-fat cappuccino		OPTION 2 – 100 g chicken, 80 g burghul: Harissa Chicken with Tabouli (see p 223)

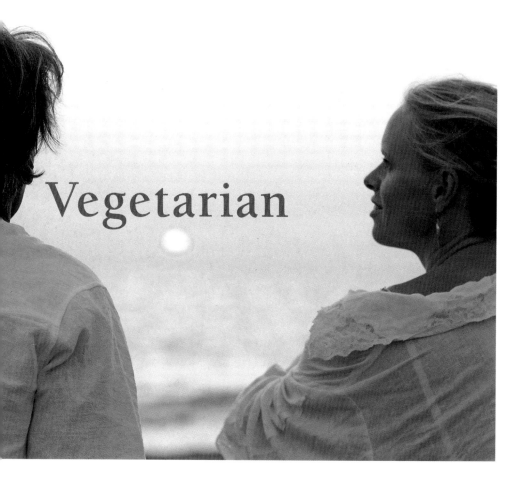

Vegetarian

DAILY SNACK

Choose from these snack options each day. You *must* at the 2 fruit units and the 1 dairy unit each day to ensure your daily food allowance is complete. Add the 1 unit nuts even if nuts are included in the menu plan for that day.

- tea or coffee with low-fat milk
- 200 g low-fat yoghurt (1 unit dairy)
- 300 g fresh fruit (2 units fruit)
- 20 g dry-roasted, unsalted nuts (1 unit nuts)

Vegetarian	Breakfast	Lunch	Dinner
Monday	40 g high-soluble-fibre cereal (e.g. Kellogg's Guardian) with 250 ml low-fat sterol milk	Roasted Carrot, Tofu & Fennel Salad (see p 160) 2 wholegrain crisp bread with 2 tsp sterol spread	OPTION 2 – 100 g legumes, 80 g cooked pasta: Tomato & Oregano Cannelloni (see p 206) 1½ cups mixed salad vegetables
Tuesday	40 g instant oats with 250 ml low-fat sterol milk	Egg & salad sandwich (2 slices wholegrain bread with 2 tsp sterol spread, 1 hard-boiled egg, 2 tsp fat-free mayonnaise, sliced spring onion & ½ cup salad leaves)	150 g legumes: Vegetable Moussaka (see p 176) 1 cup green salad with 2 tsp olive oil & a little balsamic vinegar
Wednesday	40 g unsweetened untoasted muesli with 12 g nuts & 250 ml low-fat sterol milk	Vegie Burger with Herb Aïoli (see p 158), the patty cooked in 2 tsp sterol spread	OPTION 2 – 100 g tofu, 80 g noodles: substitute tofu for chicken in Sesame Chicken with Soba Noodles & Plum Sauce (see p 224)
Thursday	40 g high-soluble-fibre cereal (e.g. Uncle Tobys Healthwise) with 250 ml low-fat sterol milk	Carrot & Ginger Soup (see p 168) 100 g salt-reduced baked beans on 1 slice wholegrain bread spread with 2 tsp sterol spread	OPTION 2 – 100 g TVP, 40 g bread: Vegetable Samosa Parcels (see p 208) 1 cup green salad drizzled with 2 tsp sesame oil
Friday	40 g unsweetened toasted muesli with 12 g nuts & 250 ml low-fat sterol milk	Curried egg sandwich (2 slices wholegrain bread with 2 tsp sterol spread, curried egg – 1 egg mashed with 2 tsp fat-free mayonnaise, low-salt curry powder and lemon juice – ½ cup watercress & sliced cucumber)	OPTION 2 – 100 g legumes, 40 g bread: Baked Beans (see p 206) 2 cups green salad with fat-free dressing
Saturday	40 g instant oats with 12 g nuts & 250 ml low-fat sterol milk	Baked beans on toast (140 g salt-reduced baked beans on 1 slice toasted wholegrain bread spread with 2 tsp sterol spread) 1 cup mixed salad vegetables with fat-free dressing	150 g tofu: 150 g tofu stir-fried in 1 tsp sesame oil with 2 cups chopped mixed vegetables
Sunday	**BRUNCH** Pea, Leek & Mint Frittata (see p 154) 1 low-fat latte or low-fat cappuccino		OPTION 2 – 100 g legumes, 80 g bread: Curried Sweet Potato Cakes (see p 208) 1 cup green salad with 2 tsp olive oil & a little balsamic vinegar 1 slice crusty wholegrain bread with 1 tsp sterol spread

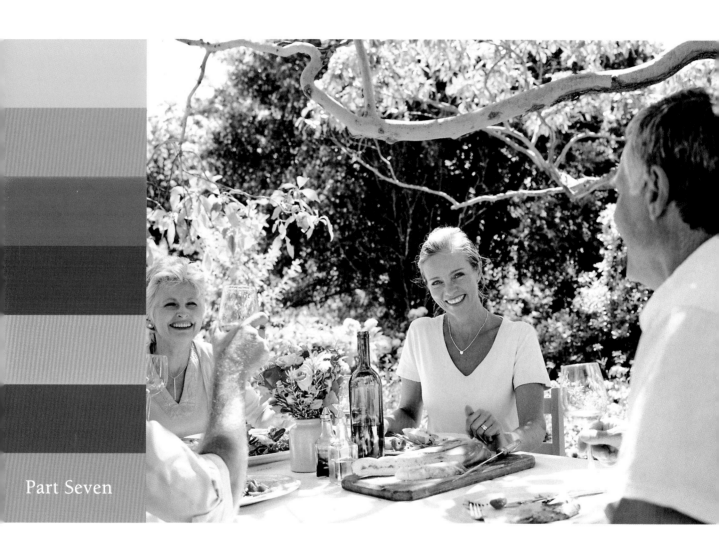

Part Seven

CLIP recipes

by Heidi Flett

Brunch

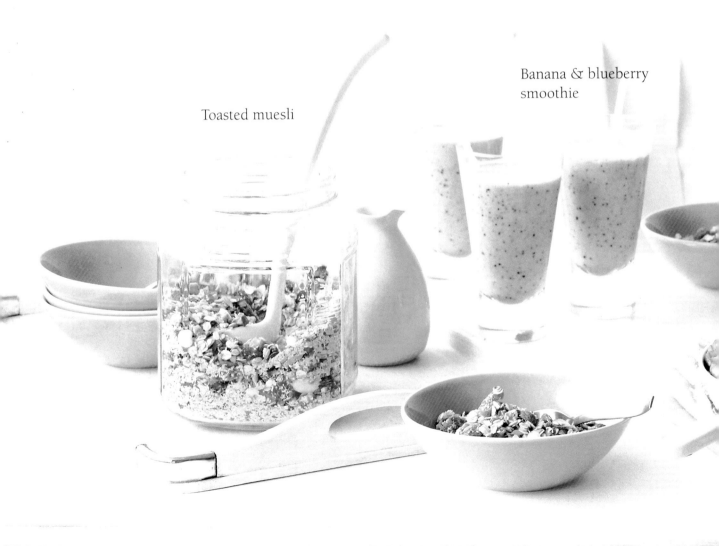

Toasted muesli

Banana & blueberry
smoothie

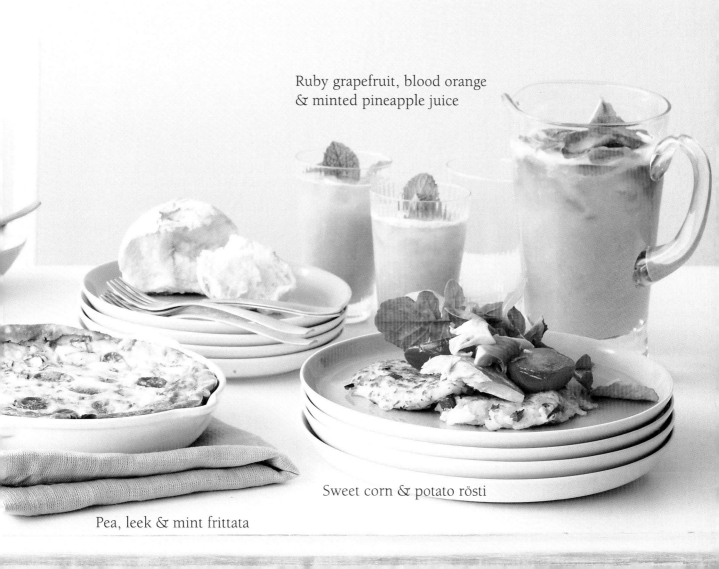

Ruby grapefruit, blood orange
& minted pineapple juice

Sweet corn & potato rösti

Pea, leek & mint frittata

Ruby grapefruit, blood orange & minted pineapple juice

350 ml ruby grapefruit juice

1 small pineapple, peeled, cored and chopped

350 ml freshly squeezed orange juice

3 blood oranges, segmented

1 tablespoon chopped mint

crushed ice

Place the grapefruit juice and pineapple in a food processor and whiz until smooth. Pour into a large serving jug and add the orange juice and segments. Stir in the mint and fill the jug with ice. Mix well and serve.

1 serve = 1½ units fruit

Pea, leek & mint frittata

1 tablespoon olive oil

1 leek, white part only, finely sliced

8 eggs

100 g low-fat ricotta

⅓ cup low-fat natural yoghurt

2 tablespoons chopped mint

150 g cherry tomatoes, halved

⅔ cup frozen peas

⅓ cup grated low-fat cheddar

1 tablespoon sterol spread

4 crusty wholegrain bread rolls

Preheat the oven to 170°C.

Heat the olive oil in a non-stick frying pan over low heat and cook the leek for 3 minutes or until softened. Transfer to a bowl and leave to cool.

Whisk together the eggs, ricotta and yoghurt, and season with freshly ground black pepper. Stir in the mint, tomatoes, peas, cheddar and leek.

Melt the sterol spread in a 20 cm ovenproof non-stick frying pan over medium heat. Add the egg mixture, stir with a spatula and cook for 5 minutes until golden underneath and nearly set. Transfer to the oven and cook for 20 minutes until golden and puffed.

Cut into wedges and serve warm with crusty bread rolls and a mixed leaf salad.

1 serve = 1 unit protein, 2 units carbohydrates, 1 unit cheese, 2 units vegetables, 1 unit fats

Banana & blueberry smoothie

600 ml low-fat sterol milk

4 ripe bananas

½ cup frozen blueberries

⅓ cup oat bran

400 g low-fat sterol vanilla or fruit yoghurt

Place all the ingredients in a blender and whiz until smooth. Pour into four tall glasses and serve immediately.

1 serve = 1 unit dairy, 1 unit fruit

Note: If you wish, replace the banana and blueberries with strawberries, mango, peach, raspberries or any other fruit you like.

Sweet corn & potato rösti with smoked trout & roasted tomatoes

4 desiree potatoes (or sweet potatoes), peeled

⅓ cup fresh or salt-reduced tinned corn kernels

½ red capsicum, finely diced

2 spring onions (scallions), finely sliced

1½ tablespoons roughly chopped coriander

1½ tablespoons roughly chopped basil

1½ tablespoons canola oil

4 Roma tomatoes, halved lengthways

olive oil spray

400 g smoked trout

Preheat the oven to 200°C and line a baking tray with baking paper.

Place the potatoes in a large saucepan of cold water, bring to the boil, then reduce the heat and simmer for 10 minutes. Drain well and cool slightly.

Coarsely grate the potatoes. Transfer to a bowl and mix with the corn, capsicum, spring onion, coriander and basil.

Heat the canola oil in a large ovenproof non-stick frying pan over medium heat. Spoon the potato mixture into the pan and cook for 5 minutes or until golden. Transfer to the oven and bake for 15 minutes or until golden and crisp.

Meanwhile, place the tomatoes on the prepared baking tray and lightly spray with olive oil. Bake for 10 minutes or until the tomatoes are soft.

Cut the rösti into wedges and serve with the roasted tomatoes and smoked trout.

1 serve = 1 unit protein, 1 unit carbohydrates, 1 unit vegetables, 2 units fats

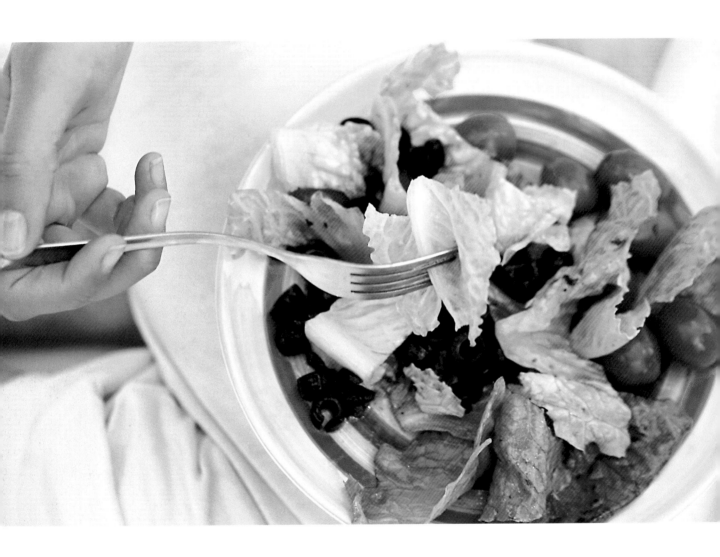

Lunches

Vegie burger with herb aïoli

Lunch Serves 4

160 g Sanitarium Vegie Delights Mince
½ red onion, finely chopped
2 tablespoons roughly chopped flat-leaf parsley
½ teaspoon ground cumin
2 gherkins, roughly chopped
1 teaspoon finely grated lemon zest
1 egg white, lightly beaten
canola oil spray
½ butter lettuce, leaves washed and separated
2 tomatoes, finely sliced
4 wholegrain bread rolls, cut in half

Herb aïoli

150 g fat-free mayonnaise
50 g low-fat natural yoghurt
2 cloves garlic, crushed
2 tablespoons lemon juice
2 tablespoons finely chopped basil
1 tablespoon finely chopped flat-leaf parsley

Place the Vegie Mince, onion, parsley, cumin, gherkins, lemon zest and egg white in a food processor and pulse until just combined. Shape the mixture into four patties, transfer to a plate, then cover and refrigerate for 20 minutes.

To make the aïoli, combine all ingredients in a bowl. Season with freshly ground black pepper.

Spray a non-stick frying pan with canola oil. Cook the patties for 3 minutes each side or until golden and cooked to your liking. To serve, place the lettuce and tomato slices on one half of each roll. Top with a patty and some aïoli and finish with the lid.

1 serve = ½ unit protein, 2 units carbohydrates,
1½ units vegetables, 1 unit fats

Smoked trout salad with orange, green beans & horseradish

Lunch Serves 4

100 g green beans, trimmed
160 g hot-smoked ocean trout, flaked
1 orange, segmented
1 avocado, peeled and diced
1 small red onion, finely sliced
100 g rocket
4 slices wholegrain bread

Horseradish dressing

¼ cup low-fat natural yoghurt
2 teaspoons grated fresh horseradish or salt-reduced prepared horseradish
1 tablespoon lemon juice

Bring a small saucepan of water to the boil, add the beans and blanch for 1 minute or until bright green and crisp. Refresh under cold running water.

Combine the trout, orange, avocado, onion, rocket and beans in a large bowl.

To make the horseradish dressing, mix together the yoghurt, horseradish and lemon juice. Drizzle over the salad and toss gently. Divide among four serving dishes and serve with bread.

1 serve = ½ unit protein, 1 unit carbohydrates,
½ unit vegetables, 3 units fats

Notes: Because this recipe is relatively high in salt, you should make it an occasional indulgence rather than a regular meal. Hot-smoked ocean trout is available in 160 g portions in the smoked salmon section of most supermarkets.

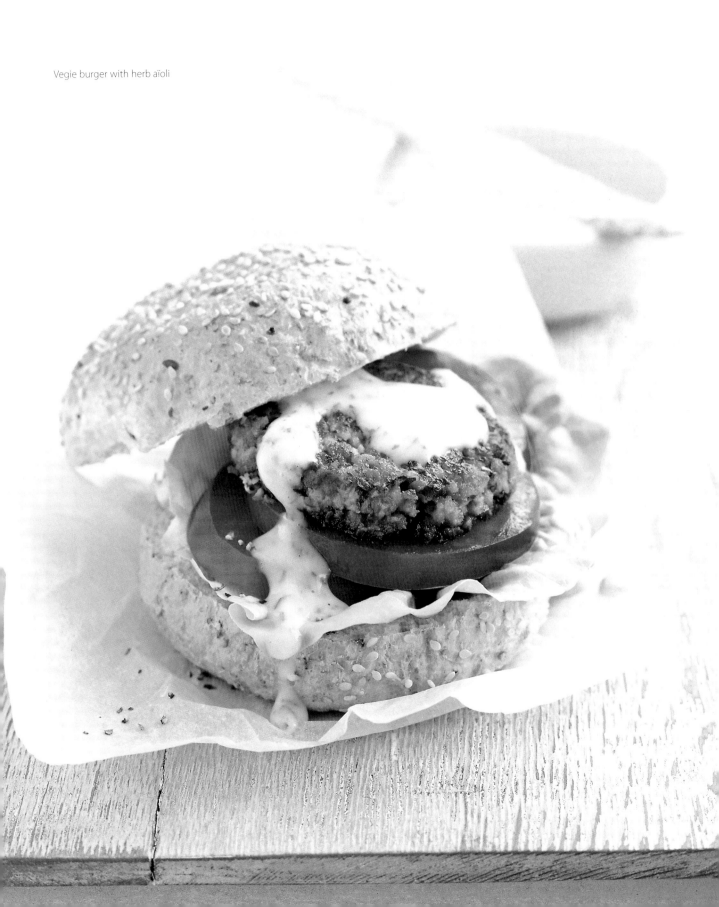

Vegie burger with herb aïoli

Bruschetta with hummus, roasted vegetables & basil

Lunch Serves 4

3 zucchini, sliced into ribbons with
    a vegetable peeler
1 red capsicum, sliced
1 yellow capsicum, sliced
1 red onion, cut into thin wedges
1 clove garlic, crushed
1 tablespoon olive oil
½ cup basil, roughly torn
8 slices wholegrain bread, toasted
160 g low-fat hummus
rocket, to serve

Preheat the oven to 200°C.

Place the zucchini, capsicum, onion and garlic in a baking dish, drizzle with olive oil and toss to coat. Roast for 10 minutes or until the vegetables are soft. Stir in the basil.

Top each slice of toast with hummus and some of the roasted vegetable mix. Serve with rocket leaves.

1 serve = ½ unit protein, 2 units carbohydrates,
1½ units vegetables, 1 unit fats

Roasted carrot, tofu & fennel salad

Lunch Serves 4

2 bunches baby carrots, trimmed and peeled
2 small red onions, cut into thin wedges
2 bulbs fennel, cut into thin wedges
2 teaspoons ground cumin
2 teaspoons ground cinnamon
1 tablespoon lemon juice
1 clove garlic, crushed
1 tablespoon brown sugar
1 tablespoon rice-wine vinegar
2 tablespoons olive oil
160 g firm tofu, cut into 2 cm dice
1 × 400 g tin salt-reduced cannellini beans, rinsed
    and drained
¼ cup coriander leaves
2 tablespoons unsalted pistachio kernels, lightly
    toasted and roughly chopped

Preheat the oven to 200°C. Combine the carrots, onion and fennel in a large ceramic baking dish.

In a small bowl, whisk together the cumin, cinnamon, lemon juice, garlic, brown sugar, vinegar and 1 tablespoon of the olive oil. Drizzle over the vegetables and roast for 30 minutes or until the carrots are tender.

Heat the remaining oil in a large non-stick frying pan over medium heat. Add the tofu and cook for 1–2 minutes or until golden on each side.

Divide the roasted vegetables among four shallow serving dishes, top with tofu and cannellini beans and sprinkle with coriander and pistachios.

1 serve = ½ unit protein, 1 unit carbohydrates,
1½ units vegetables, 3 units fats

Roasted carrot, tofu & fennel salad

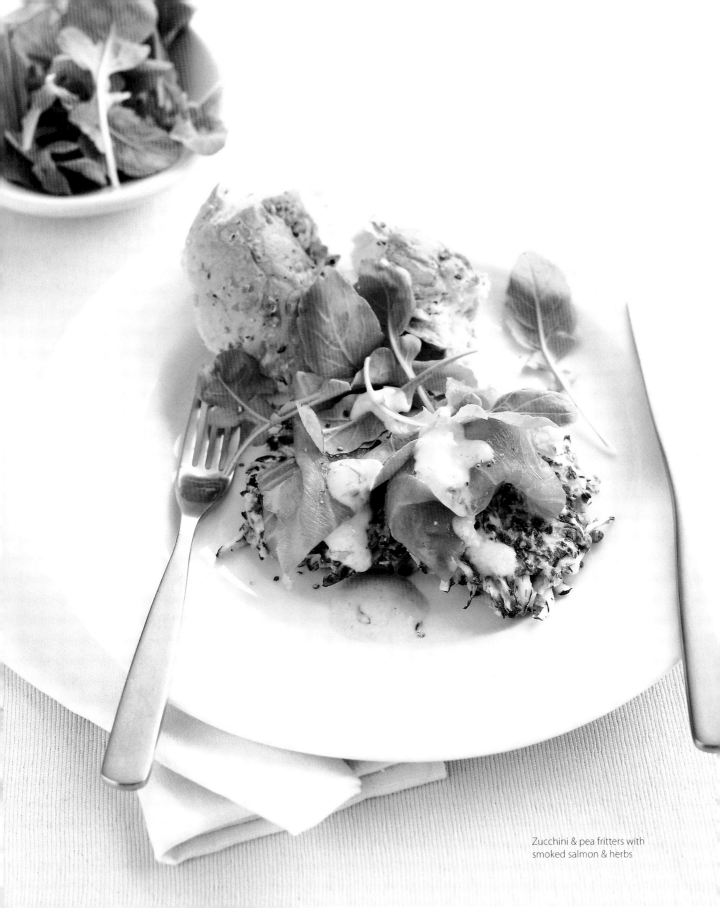

Zucchini & pea fritters with
smoked salmon & herbs

Zucchini & pea fritters with smoked salmon & herbs

Lunch Serves 4

4 zucchini, grated

2 spring onions (scallions) , finely sliced

½ cup wholemeal plain flour

2 teaspoons finely grated lemon zest

½ cup frozen peas, thawed, crushed with a fork

2 eggs, lightly beaten

2 tablespoons roughly chopped dill

2 tablespoons roughly chopped mint

canola oil spray

4 slices smoked salmon, halved

rocket or baby spinach leaves, to serve

4 wholegrain bread rolls

Lemon yoghurt dressing

½ cup low-fat natural yoghurt

2 tablespoons finely shredded mint

1 teaspoon ground cumin

1 teaspoon finely grated lemon zest

2 tablespoons lemon juice

To make the dressing, place all the ingredients in a bowl and mix well. Set aside.

Combine the zucchini, spring onion, flour, zest, peas, egg, dill and mint in a bowl. Season with freshly ground black pepper.

Heat a large non-stick frying pan over medium heat and lightly spray with canola oil. Add ¼-cup scoops of mixture to make eight fritters and cook for 3–4 minutes each side, until golden and cooked through. Top each fritter with smoked salmon and drizzle with dressing. Serve with rocket or spinach leaves and a wholegrain bread roll.

1 serve = ½ unit protein, 2 units carbohydrates,
1 unit vegetables

Pizza with tomato, artichoke & mushrooms

Lunch Serves 4

2 × 26 cm wholemeal Lebanese flatbreads

200 g salt-reduced tomato pasta sauce

125 g low-fat pizza cheese

100 g marinated artichokes, drained and sliced

200 g cherry tomatoes, halved

200 g Swiss brown mushrooms, sliced

160 g salt-reduced ham, roughly chopped

2 teaspoons dried oregano

baby rocket, to serve

Preheat the oven to 220°C. Place the flatbread on two baking trays and spread with the pasta sauce, leaving a thin border around the edge. Sprinkle with half the cheese, then top with the artichoke, tomato, mushroom, ham and oregano. Sprinkle with the remaining cheese.

Bake for 15 minutes or until the cheese is golden and the bases are crisp. Remove from the oven, top with rocket leaves and serve immediately.

1 serve = ½ unit protein, 2 units carbohydrates,
1 unit cheese, 1½ units vegetables

Pita bread, tomato & tuna salad

Lunch Serves 4

4 small wholemeal pita breads

olive oil spray

160 g tuna tinned in spring water, drained

2 spring onions (scallions), finely sliced

2 Lebanese cucumbers, finely sliced

2 vine-ripened tomatoes, diced

2 baby cos lettuce, leaves separated and torn

2 tablespoons roughly chopped flat-leaf parsley

2 tablespoons roughly chopped mint

50 g pitted black olives, chopped

Lemon vinaigrette

2 tablespoons olive oil

1 tablespoon lemon juice

1 teaspoon dried oregano

1 teaspoon Dijon mustard

Preheat the oven to 200°C. Tear the pita bread into 4 cm pieces, place on a baking tray and lightly spray with olive oil. Bake for 5 minutes or until golden and crisp.

To make the vinaigrette, place all the ingredients in a screw-top jar and shake until well combined.

Mix together the tuna, spring onion, cucumber, tomato, lettuce, parsley, mint and olives in a large bowl. Drizzle the dressing over the top, add the pita chips and toss gently to combine.

1 serve = ½ unit protein, 2 units carbohydrates, 1½ units vegetables, 2 units fats

Chicken, snow pea & pumpkin salad

Lunch Serves 4

300 g butternut pumpkin, peeled and cut
    into 2 cm chunks

1 tablespoon olive oil

160 g smoked skinless chicken breast, thinly sliced

125 g snow peas, trimmed and sliced on an angle

250 g cherry tomatoes, halved

2 tablespoons roughly chopped tarragon

100 g baby spinach leaves

2 cups green beans, trimmed, blanched
    and refreshed

1 × 400 g tin salt-reduced cannellini beans, rinsed
    and drained

1 tablespoon flaked almonds, lightly toasted

4 slices wholegrain bread

Vinaigrette

2 tablespoons olive oil

2 teaspoons red-wine vinegar

2 teaspoons Dijon mustard

1 clove garlic, crushed

Preheat the oven to 200°C. Place the pumpkin in a baking dish and toss with the olive oil. Bake for 30 minutes or until tender. Remove from the oven and allow to cool slightly.

To make the vinaigrette, whisk together the olive oil, vinegar, mustard and garlic.

Combine the pumpkin, chicken, snow peas, tomatoes, tarragon, spinach, green beans, cannellini beans and almonds in a large bowl. Pour dressing over salad and toss well. Divide among four serving plates and serve with bread.

1 serve = ½ unit protein, 2 units carbohydrates, 2 units vegetables, 2 units fats

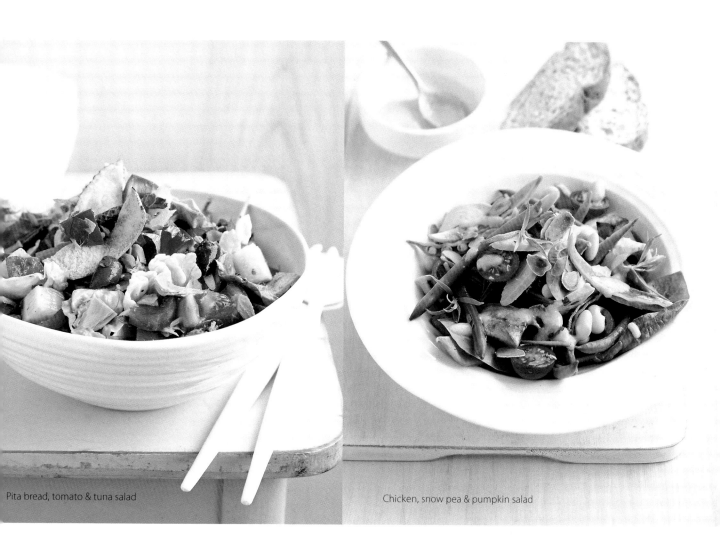

Pita bread, tomato & tuna salad

Chicken, snow pea & pumpkin salad

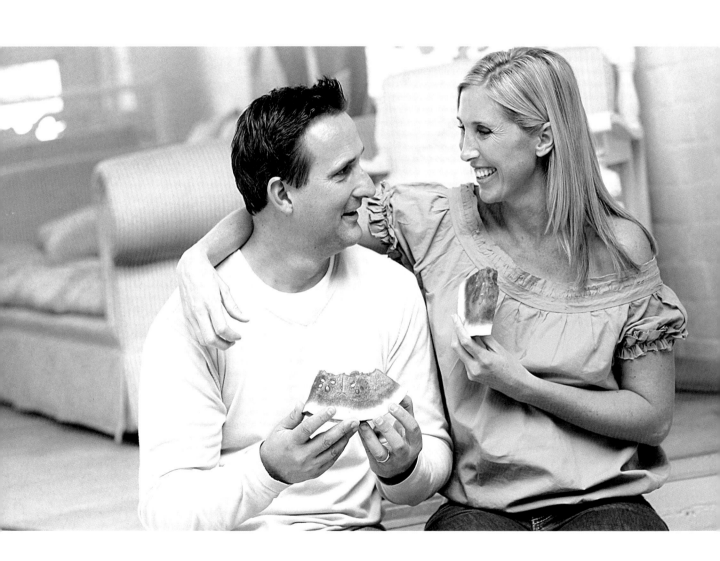

Snacks

Hot & sour pumpkin soup

Free

- ¼ cup tom yum paste
- 1 litre salt-reduced chicken stock
- 400 g butternut pumpkin, peeled and cut into 2 cm chunks
- 1 tomato, seeded and diced
- 100 g snow peas, finely sliced
- juice of 1 lime
- ½ cup coriander leaves, roughly chopped, plus extra to garnish
- 2 spring onions (scallions), finely sliced on an angle

Combine the tom yum paste and stock in a large heavy-based saucepan and bring to the boil. Reduce the heat to medium.

Add the pumpkin and simmer for 6–8 minutes or until the pumpkin is just tender. Add the tomato and snow peas and simmer for 5 minutes.

Stir in the lime juice, coriander and spring onion. Ladle into bowls or mugs and garnish with the extra coriander leaves.

Carrot & ginger soup

Free

- 1 tablespoon olive oil
- 1 large onion, finely sliced
- 8 carrots, peeled and chopped
- 4 teaspoons crushed ginger
- 2 cloves garlic, crushed
- 1 long red chilli, seeded and finely sliced
- 1 teaspoon finely grated orange zest
- 1 litre salt-reduced vegetable stock
- ¼ cup roughly chopped coriander
- 4 tablespoons low-fat natural yoghurt

Heat the oil in a large heavy-based saucepan over medium heat. Add the onion and cook for 2–3 minutes or until soft.

Add the carrot, ginger, garlic, chilli and orange zest and cook for 5 minutes or until the vegetables start to soften. Add the stock and bring to the boil, then reduce the heat and simmer, covered, for 15 minutes or until the carrots are very tender. Remove from the heat.

Allow to cool for 15–20 minutes, then spoon the soup into a blender, or use a stick blender, and whiz until smooth (thin it out with extra vegetable stock or water if necessary). Return the soup to the pan and bring to a simmer. Stir in the coriander, ladle into bowls or mugs and serve with a dollop of yoghurt.

Hot & sour pumpkin soup

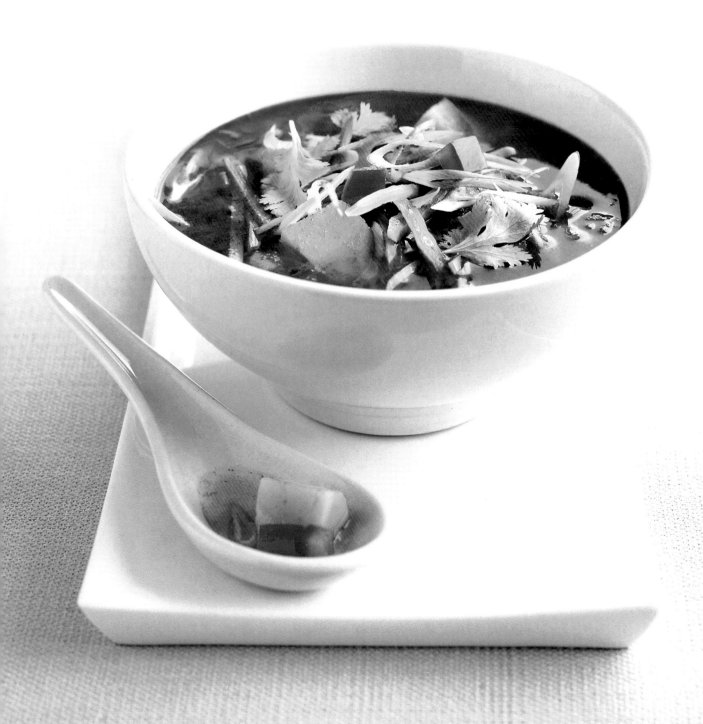

Dips

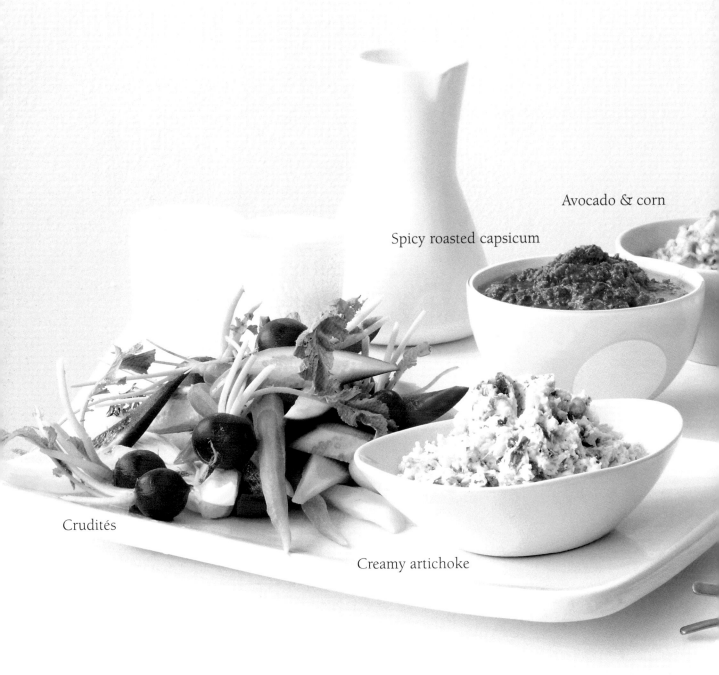

Avocado & corn

Spicy roasted capsicum

Crudités

Creamy artichoke

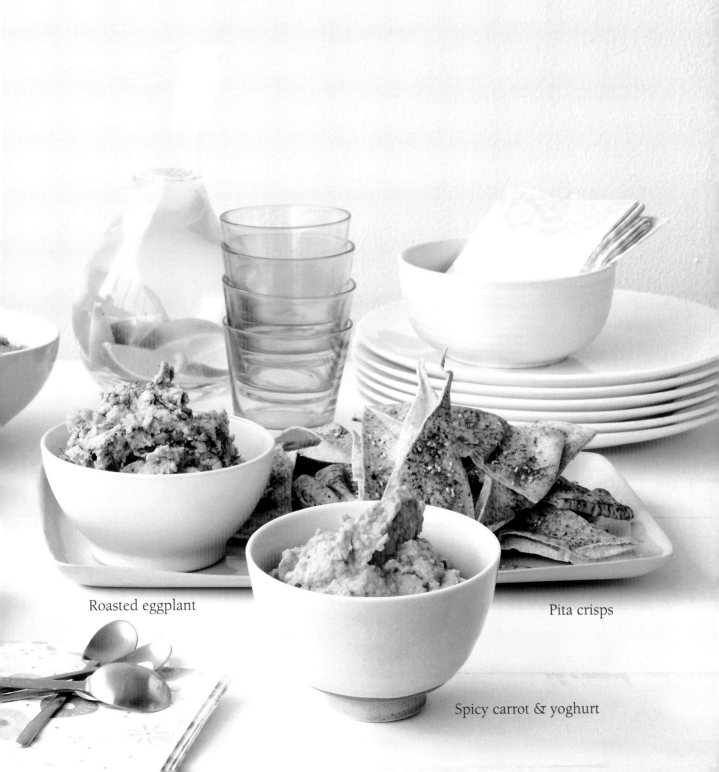

Roasted eggplant

Pita crisps

Spicy carrot & yoghurt

Avocado & corn dip

Serves 4–6

- 1 ripe avocado, peeled
- 1 small red onion, finely chopped
- 1 green chilli, seeded and finely chopped
- juice of 1 lime
- ½ cup roughly chopped coriander
- 1 × 250 g tin salt-reduced corn kernels, drained
- 2 tomatoes, diced
- 1 Lebanese cucumber, seeded and finely diced

Place the avocado, onion, chilli, lime juice and coriander in a food processor and pulse until combined. Fold in the corn, tomato and cucumber.

1 serve = 2 units fats

Spicy roasted capsicum dip

Free Serves 4–6

- 1 × 450 g jar roasted red capsicums, drained
- 1 teaspoon sambal oelek, or to taste
- 2 cloves garlic, roughly chopped
- 2 teaspoons ground cumin
- 1 red onion, finely diced
- ¼ cup lemon juice
- ½ cup low-fat natural yoghurt

Place all the ingredients in a food processor and whiz until smooth.

Creamy artichoke dip

Serves 4–6

- 1 × 340 g jar marinated artichokes, drained
- 1 clove garlic, roughly chopped
- 2 tablespoons lemon juice
- 3 tablespoons low-fat ricotta
- 3 spring onions (scallions), finely sliced
- 2 tablespoons roughly chopped flat-leaf parsley

Place the artichokes, garlic, lemon juice and ricotta in a food processor and whiz until smooth. Fold in the spring onion and parsley and season well with freshly ground black pepper.

1 serve = 1 unit fats

Roasted eggplant dip

Serves 4–6

- 2 eggplants, cut into 3 cm dice
- olive oil spray
- 2 cloves garlic, roughly chopped
- 2 tablespoons tahini
- 3 spring onions (scallions), roughly chopped
- ¼ cup lemon juice
- 1 teaspoon ground cumin
- ⅓ cup roughly chopped coriander

Preheat the oven to 200°C. Place the eggplant on a baking tray, lightly spray with olive oil and roast for 15 minutes or until soft and golden. Place the eggplant and remaining ingredients in a food processor and pulse until combined. Season with freshly ground black pepper.

1 serve = 2 units fats

Spicy carrot & yoghurt dip

Free Serves 4–6

> 1 tablespoon olive oil
> 2 cups frozen carrot slices, thawed
> 1 small red onion, roughly chopped
> ½ teaspoon ground cinnamon
> ¼ teaspoon chilli powder
> 2 tablespoons lemon juice
> ⅓ cup low-fat natural yoghurt
> 1 tablespoon roughly chopped flat-leaf parsley
> 2 tablespoons roughly chopped coriander

Heat the oil a large non-stick frying pan over medium heat and cook the carrot and onion for 2 minutes or until the onion has softened. Add the cinnamon and chilli powder and cook for 30 seconds.

Place the carrot mixture in a food processor with the lemon juice and yoghurt and whiz until smooth. Fold in the herbs.

Crudités

Free

> assorted vegetables, such as carrots, radishes, celery, cucumber or red or yellow capsicum

Cut the vegetables into sticks or chunks and arrange them in piles on a serving platter. Serve with your choice of dips.

Pita crisps

Serves 4

> 2 large wholemeal pita breads
> olive oil spray
> 1 tablespoon dukkah

Preheat the oven to 200°C and line a baking tray with baking paper.

Spray the pita breads with olive oil and sprinkle with dukkah. Cut each bread into eight wedges and place on the baking tray. Bake for 5–10 minutes or until golden brown and crisp. Serve with your choice of dips.

1 serve = 1 unit carbohydrates

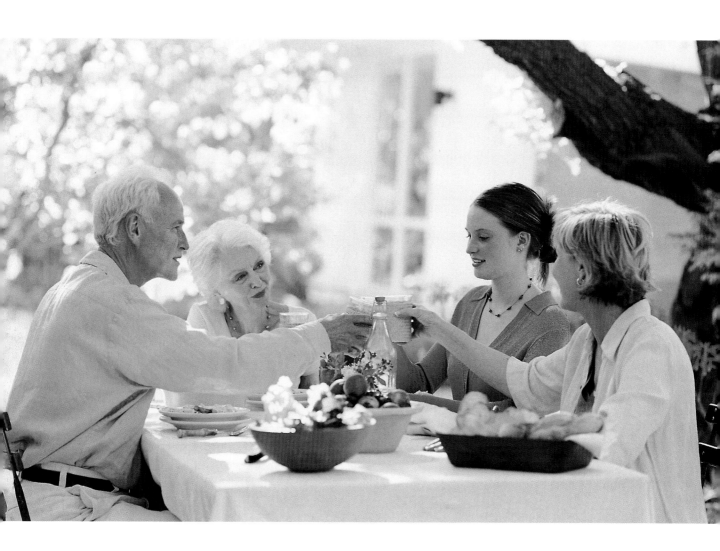

Dinners

Option 1

Chargrilled beef with zucchini, pine nuts & spinach

Dinner Serves 4

600 g rump steak, trimmed
canola oil spray
olive oil spray
3 zucchini, finely sliced lengthways
200 g cherry tomatoes, halved
1 small red onion, finely sliced
1 tablespoon lemon juice
1 tablespoon pine nuts
150 g baby spinach leaves, finely
   shredded
¼ cup roughly torn mint

Cumin yoghurt
½ teaspoon ground cumin
200 ml low-fat natural yoghurt
1 Lebanese cucumber, seeded and
   coarsely grated
1 tablespoon lemon juice

Preheat a chargrill or barbecue grill to very hot. Lightly spray the steak with canola oil and cook for 3 minutes each side for medium or until cooked to your liking. Transfer to a plate, cover lightly with foil and allow to rest for 5 minutes.

Preheat a large non-stick frying pan over medium heat, lightly spray with olive oil and cook the zucchini for 1 minute. Add the tomatoes, onion and lemon juice and cook for 2 minutes or until the tomatoes are softened and heated through. Season with freshly ground black pepper and cool slightly.

Place the pine nuts, spinach and mint in a large bowl, then stir in the zucchini mixture.

To make the cumin yoghurt, place all the ingredients in a small bowl and mix well.

To serve, spoon the zucchini mixture onto a large serving plate or platter. Thickly slice the beef and lay it over the vegetables. Drizzle with the cumin yoghurt and serve with a salad.

1 serve = 1½ units protein, 1½ units vegetables

Fish & vegetable skewers

Dinner Serves 4

600 g firm white fish (barramundi, gemfish
    or flathead)
1 teaspoon dried oregano
1 clove garlic, crushed
1 tablespoon olive oil
2 teaspoons lemon juice
16 cherry tomatoes
2 zucchini, halved lengthways and cut
    into 2 cm slices
2 red onions, cut into thin wedges
1 yellow capsicum, seeded and cut into
    2 cm pieces
lemon wedges

If using bamboo skewers, soak them in cold water for
30 minutes before use (you'll need eight).

Cut the fish into 4 cm pieces, place in a small bowl with
the oregano, garlic, olive oil and lemon juice and stir to
combine. Cover and leave to marinate for a few minutes.

Preheat a chargrill or barbecue grill to high. Onto each
skewer thread a cherry tomato, and pieces of zucchini,
onion, fish and capsicum, then repeat to finish the skewer.
Place on the grill and cook for 5 minutes each side or until
lightly charred and the fish is cooked through. Serve with
lemon wedges and a leafy salad.

1 serve = 1½ units protein, 2 units vegetables, 1 unit fats

Chargrilled squid salad

Dinner Serves 4

600 g squid tubes, finely sliced into rings
2 tablespoons lime juice
1 teaspoon dried marjoram
1 large red chilli, seeded and finely chopped
12 cherry tomatoes, quartered
2 roasted red capsicums, finely sliced (buy in jars)
½ cup roughly torn basil
1 tablespoon red-wine vinegar
2 tablespoons olive oil
2 baby cos lettuce leaves, torn
lime wedges

Place the squid, lime juice, marjoram and chilli in a bowl
and mix well. Cover and leave to marinate in the fridge
for a few minutes.

Combine the tomatoes, capsicum and basil in a large
bowl and drizzle with the vinegar and olive oil. Add the
cos leaves.

Preheat a chargrill or barbecue grill to high. When the
plate is very hot, cook the squid for 2–3 minutes, then
add to the salad and toss well to combine. Serve with
lime wedges.

1 serve = 1½ units protein, 2 units vegetables, 2 units fats

Prawn & cucumber salad with mango

Dinner Serves 4

2 Lebanese cucumbers, sliced into ribbons
   with a vegetable peeler
1 cup bean sprouts
2 spring onions (scallions), finely sliced on an angle
600 g cooked, peeled and deveined king prawns,
   tails intact
2 tablespoons roughly chopped mint
2 tablespoons roughly chopped Vietnamese mint
¼ cup roughly chopped coriander
50 g snow pea sprouts
1 mango, peeled and sliced

Dressing
juice and finely grated zest of 1 lime
1 tablespoon low-salt soy sauce
1 teaspoon brown sugar
2 tablespoons olive oil
1 long red chilli, finely chopped (optional)

To make the dressing, place all the dressing ingredients
in a screw-top jar and shake until well combined.

Place all the salad ingredients in a large mixing bowl.
Drizzle the dressing over the salad, toss everything together
and divide among serving plates.

1 serve = 1½ units protein, 2 units vegetables, 2 units fats

Prawn & tomato soup with mussels

Dinner Serves 4

1 tablespoon olive oil
1 onion, finely chopped
2 sticks celery, finely diced
2 cloves garlic, crushed
1 long red chilli, finely sliced
½ teaspoon dried oregano
1 × 400 g tin salt-reduced chopped tomatoes
1 cup white wine
3 cups salt-reduced chicken stock
400 g uncooked prawns, peeled and deveined,
   tails intact
1 kg mussels, scrubbed and debearded
1 bunch asparagus, cut into 2 cm pieces
100 g snow peas, sliced in half on an angle
¼ cup roughly chopped flat-leaf parsley
1 tablespoon finely grated lemon zest

Heat the oil in a large heavy-based saucepan over medium
heat and cook the onion, celery, garlic, chilli and oregano
for 2–3 minutes or until soft. Add the tomatoes, wine and
stock, bring to the boil, then reduce the heat and simmer
for 15 minutes.

Add the prawns, asparagus, snow peas and mussels
and simmer, covered, for 5 minutes or until the prawns are
cooked through, the mussels are open and the asparagus
and snow peas are just cooked. Stir in the parsley and
lemon zest and ladle into serving bowls.

1 serve = 1½ units protein, 2 units vegetables, 1 unit fats

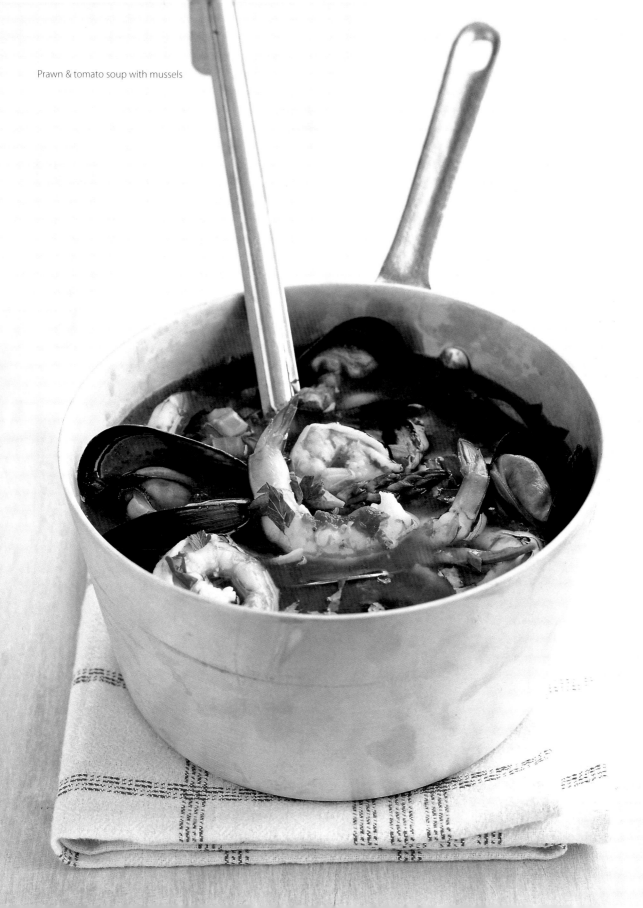

Prawn & tomato soup with mussels

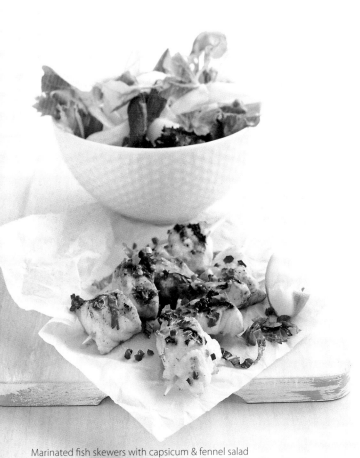

Marinated fish skewers with capsicum & fennel salad

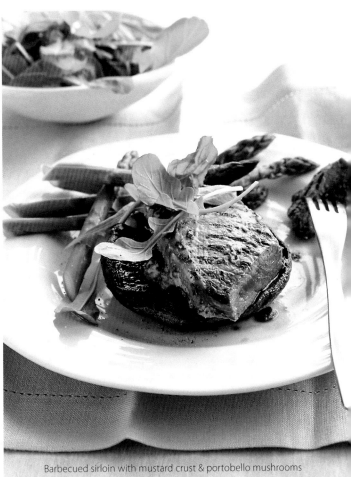

Barbecued sirloin with mustard crust & portobello mushrooms

Marinated fish skewers with capsicum & fennel salad

Dinner Serves 4

600 g firm white fish (barramundi, gemfish or flathead)
2 teaspoons extra virgin olive oil
juice and finely grated zest of 1 lime
1 red chilli, seeded and finely chopped
¼ cup roughly chopped coriander
¼ cup roughly chopped mint
2 teaspoons coriander seeds, crushed

Capsicum & fennel salad
2 roasted red capsicums, thickly sliced (buy in jars)
1 bulb fennel, finely sliced
1 witlof, leaves separated
50 g mixed salad leaves
¼ cup olive oil
2 teaspoons balsamic vinegar

If using bamboo skewers, soak them in cold water for 30 minutes before use (you'll need eight).

Cut the fish into 4 cm pieces and thread evenly onto the skewers. Place in a ceramic dish. Whisk together the olive oil, lime juice and zest, chilli, herbs and coriander seeds in a small bowl and pour over the skewers. Cover with plastic wrap and marinate in the fridge for 20 minutes.

Preheat a chargrill or barbecue grill to medium. Cook the skewers for 3 minutes each side or until the fish is cooked through, basting with any remaining marinade.

To make the salad, combine all the vegetables in a bowl. Mix together the oil and vinegar and drizzle over the salad. Divide among four plates and serve with the fish skewers.

1 serve = 1½ units protein, 2 units vegetables, 2 units fats

Barbecued sirloin with mustard crust & portobello mushrooms

Dinner Serves 4

4 large portobello mushrooms
olive oil spray
4 × 150 g sirloin steaks, trimmed

Mustard crust
1 cup roughly torn basil
½ cup roughly torn flat-leaf parsley
¼ cup roughly torn tarragon
2 cloves garlic
2 tablespoons Dijon mustard
2 teaspoons finely grated lemon zest
2 tablespoons lemon juice

Preheat the oven to 200°C. Place the mushrooms on a baking tray, stalk-side up, and season with freshly ground black pepper. Lightly spray with olive oil, cover with foil and roast for 20 minutes or until soft.

Meanwhile, to make the mustard crust, place all the ingredients in a food processor and whiz to a smooth paste. Rub the crust into both sides of the steaks and set aside for 5 minutes.

Heat a chargrill or barbecue grill to medium. Cook the steaks for 3–4 minutes each side or until cooked to your liking. Transfer to a plate, cover lightly with foil and leave to rest for 5 minutes before serving with the mushrooms and a rocket salad or other green vegetables.

1 serve = 1½ units protein

Hot-smoked salmon, watercress & pink grapefruit salad

Dinner Serves 4

600 g hot-smoked salmon

1 bunch watercress, trimmed

2 pink grapefruit, segmented

2 Lebanese cucumbers, halved lengthways
and finely sliced

1 bulb fennel, finely sliced

2 firm pears, cored and sliced

½ avocado, peeled and sliced

Lemon vinaigrette

1 tablespoon olive oil

1 tablespoon lemon juice

1 teaspoon dried oregano

1 teaspoon Dijon mustard

To make the vinaigrette, place all the vinaigrette ingredients in a screw-top jar and shake until well combined.

Using your fingers, break the salmon into large chunks and place in a large bowl with the other salad ingredients. Drizzle with the vinaigrette and lightly toss to combine. Divide among four plates and serve.

1 serve = 1½ units protein, 1½ units vegetables,
1 unit fruit, 2 units fats

Notes: Because this recipe is relatively high in salt, you should make it an occasional indulgence rather than a regular meal. Hot smoked salmon is available in 160 g portions in the smoked salmon section of most supermarkets.

Sticky chicken drumsticks

Dinner Serves 4

8 skinless chicken drumsticks

1 teaspoon dried chilli flakes

¼ teaspoon dried rosemary

1 tablespoon smoked paprika

2 cloves garlic, crushed

1 tablespoon olive oil

juice and finely grated zest of 1 orange

juice and finely grated zest of 1 lemon

2 tablespoons honey

Place the chicken, chilli, rosemary, paprika, garlic, olive oil, orange zest and lemon zest in a large bowl. Using your hands, mix everything together, making sure the chicken is evenly coated. Cover and place in the fridge to marinate for 15–30 minutes. Preheat the oven to 180°C.

Transfer the chicken to a baking dish, cover loosely with foil and bake for 30 minutes. Remove from the oven.

Mix together the orange and lemon juices and honey and pour over the chicken.

Increase the oven temperature to 200°C and bake the chicken, basting frequently, for a further 20 minutes or until cooked through and sticky. Serve with steamed greens and carrots or a salad.

1 serve = 1½ units protein, 1 unit fats

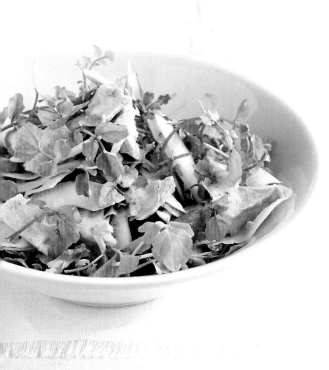
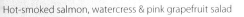

Hot-smoked salmon, watercress & pink grapefruit salad

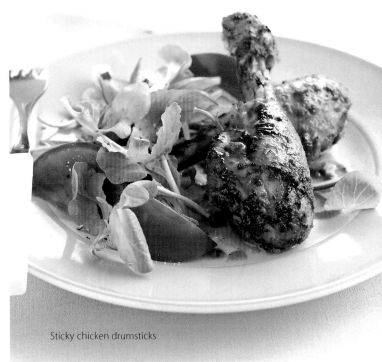

Sticky chicken drumsticks

Roasted gemfish with saffron & cardamom pumpkin

Dinner Serves 4

2 tablespoons olive oil

pinch of saffron

650 g pumpkin, peeled and cut into 3 cm chunks

1 teaspoon ground cardamom

olive oil spray

4 × 150 g gemfish fillets

1 tablespoon sesame seeds, lightly toasted

150 g baby spinach leaves

4 spring onions (scallions), finely sliced

lime wedges

Preheat the oven to 200°C. Place the olive oil, saffron, pumpkin and cardamom in a baking dish and toss gently until the pumpkin is evenly coated. Roast for 20 minutes or until tender.

Meanwhile, lightly spray a non-stick frying pan with olive oil and place the pan over medium heat. When hot, add the gemfish fillets, flesh-side down. Cook for 4 minutes each side.

Mix the sesame seeds, spinach leaves and spring onion through the pumpkin and divide among four plates. Serve with the gemfish and lime wedges, and broccolini if desired.

1 serve = 1½ units protein, 2 units vegetables, 2 units fats

Roasted salmon salad with minted chilli dressing

Dinner Serves 4

olive oil spray

4 × 150 g salmon fillets, skin removed

1 bunch asparagus, trimmed and halved crossways

100 g snow peas, trimmed

1 bulb fennel, finely sliced

100 g mixed salad leaves

200 g cherry tomatoes, halved

Minted chilli dressing

1 long red chilli, sliced lengthways and seeded

¼ cup chopped mint

juice of 2 limes

1 teaspoon brown sugar

¼ cup olive oil

Lightly spray a non-stick frying pan with olive oil and place over medium heat. When hot, add the salmon fillets and cook for 4 minutes each side.

Meanwhile bring a saucepan of water to the boil. Add the asparagus and snow peas and blanch for 1–2 minutes or until bright green but still crisp. Drain and refresh under cold running water.

To make the dressing, place all the dressing ingredients in a screw-top jar and shake until well combined.

Place the asparagus, snow peas, fennel, salad leaves and tomatoes in a large bowl. Drizzle with half the dressing, and gently toss to combine. Divide the salad among four plates and serve with a salmon fillet and a splash of the remaining dressing.

1 serve = 1½ units protein, 2 units vegetables, 3 units fats

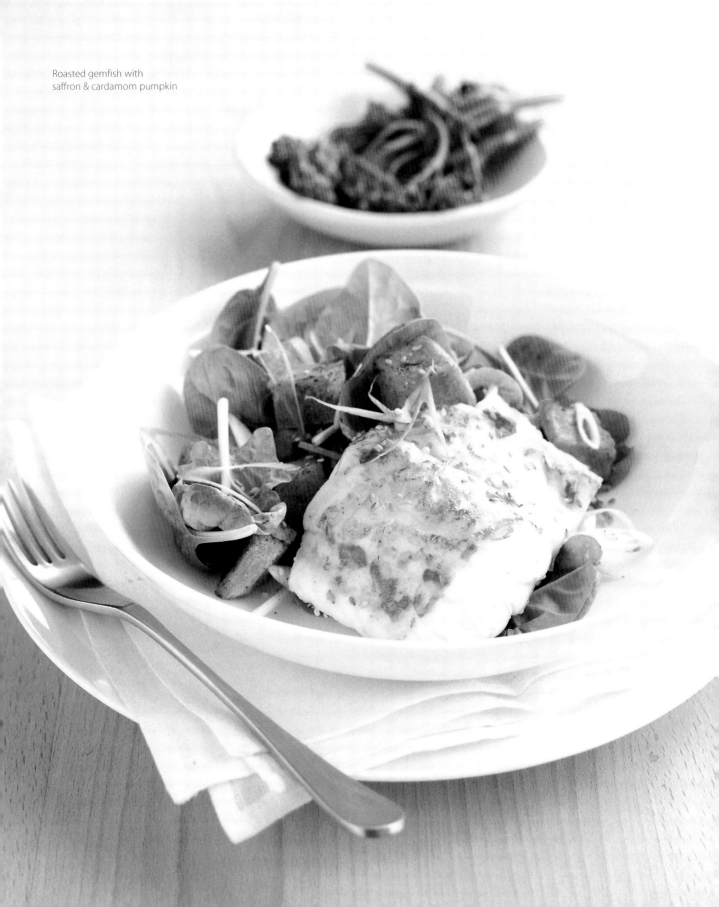

Roasted gemfish with
saffron & cardamom pumpkin

Sumac-roasted chicken with
beetroot & almond salad

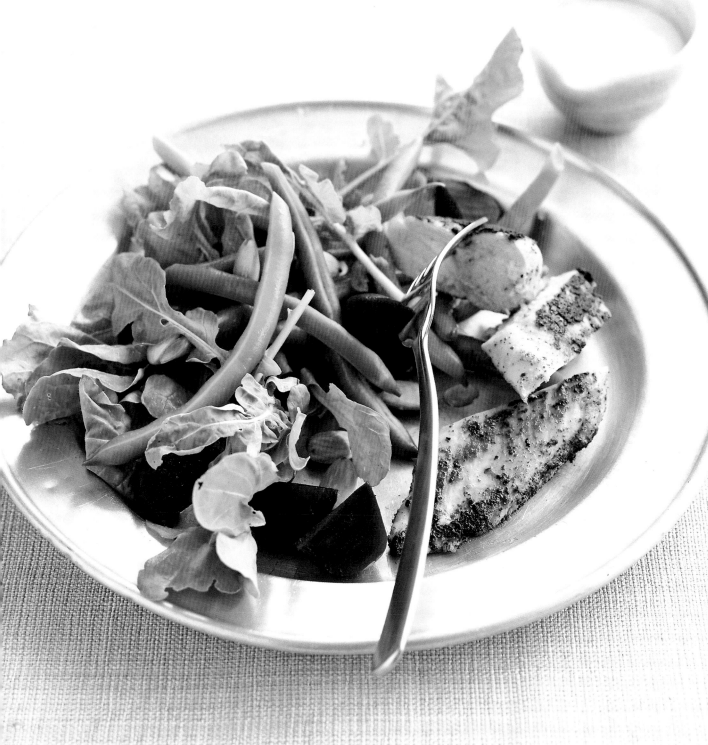

Sumac-roasted chicken with beetroot & almond salad

Dinner Serves 4

- 2 teaspoons finely grated lemon zest
- 1 clove garlic, crushed
- 2 teaspoons olive oil
- 1 tablespoon sumac
- 4 × 150 g skinless chicken breasts
- 100 g green beans, trimmed
- 1 × 450 g tin salt-reduced whole baby beetroot, drained and halved
- 2 bunches rocket
- 80 g blanched almonds, lightly toasted
- ½ cup low-fat natural yoghurt
- 2 tablespoons lemon juice

Preheat the oven to 200°C.

Combine the lemon zest, garlic, olive oil and sumac in a bowl, add the chicken breasts and rub the mixture in well. Leave to marinate for 10 minutes.

Heat a non-stick frying pan over medium heat, add the chicken breasts and cook for 2 minutes each side or until golden brown. Transfer to a baking tray, cover with foil and bake for 6–8 minutes or until cooked through.

Bring a saucepan of water to the boil, add the beans and blanch for 1 minute. Drain and refresh under cold running water.

Toss together the beetroot, rocket, almonds and beans, then divide among serving plates. Cut the chicken into thick slices and arrange next to the salad. Mix together the yoghurt and lemon juice, drizzle over the salad and serve.

1 serve = 1½ units protein, 2 units vegetables,
1 unit nuts, 2 units fats

Notes: Sumac is a Middle-Eastern spice, available from specialist food shops.

Spiced chicken casserole

Dinner Serves 4

- 1 tablespoon wholemeal plain flour
- 2 teaspoons ground cumin
- ½ teaspoon dried chilli flakes (optional)
- 1 teaspoon ground turmeric
- 1 kg skinless chicken thigh cutlets (with bone)
- 2 tablespoons olive oil
- 2 onions, diced
- 3 sticks celery, sliced
- 2 cloves garlic, crushed
- 1 litre salt-reduced chicken stock
- 1 stick cinnamon
- pinch of saffron
- 200 g pumpkin, peeled and cut into 3 cm dice
- juice and finely grated zest of 1 lemon
- ¼ cup roughly chopped coriander

Preheat the oven to 170°C. Combine the flour, cumin, chilli and turmeric in a bowl. Add the chicken and toss to coat well, pressing the spiced flour into the meat.

Heat 1 tablespoon of the olive oil in a heavy-based flameproof casserole dish (with a lid) over medium heat and cook the onion, celery and garlic for 3 minutes or until softened. Remove from the pan and add the remaining oil. Add half the chicken and cook for 2 minutes or until browned. Remove from the dish and repeat with the remaining chicken.

Return the chicken and onion mixture to the dish with the stock, cinnamon, saffron and pumpkin. Bring to the boil, then cover and cook in the oven for 45 minutes.

Skim any excess fat from the surface of the casserole. Stir in the lemon juice and zest and the coriander, and serve with steamed greens.

1 serve = 1½ units protein, 1 unit vegetables, 2 units fats

Stir-fried pork with green beans & mixed mushrooms

Dinner Serves 4

2 tablespoons canola oil

600 g pork fillet, thickly sliced

2 cloves garlic, crushed

1 tablespoon finely chopped ginger

1 long green chilli, finely sliced

100 g green beans, trimmed

1 bunch broccolini, cut into 5 cm pieces

1 red capsicum, sliced

500 g mixed mushrooms (oyster, shiitake, enoki, Swiss brown)

5 spring onions (scallions), sliced on an angle

2 tablespoons oyster sauce

⅔ cup raw unsalted cashews, lightly toasted

¼ cup roughly chopped coriander

Heat a wok over high heat, add 1 tablespoon of the oil and heat until just beginning to smoke. Add half the pork and cook for 2 minutes or until browned, then remove to a bowl. Cook the remaining pork until browned, then set aside in the bowl.

Heat the remaining oil and stir-fry the garlic, ginger and chilli for 30 seconds. Add the beans, broccolini, capsicum and mushrooms and cook for 2 minutes or until the mushrooms are soft and the beans are bright green. Return the pork to the wok and stir in the spring onion and oyster sauce. Sprinkle with cashews and coriander and serve immediately.

1 serve = 1½ units protein, 2 units vegetables,
1 unit nuts, 2 units fats

Note: If you are vegetarian, replace the pork with 600 g firm tofu.

Braised pork with dried cherries

Dinner Serves 4

2 tablespoons olive oil

2 bunches spring onions (scallions), trimmed

1 bulb fennel, cut into thin wedges

2 sticks celery, roughly chopped

2 cloves garlic, crushed

1 × 400 g tin salt-reduced chopped tomatoes

1 cup red wine or salt-reduced beef stock

60 g dried cherries

600 g pork loin, trimmed and skin removed

2 tablespoons roughly chopped flat-leaf parsley

Preheat the oven to 180°C.

Heat 1 tablespoon of the oil in a large heavy-based frying pan over medium heat and cook the spring onions, fennel, celery and garlic for 8 minutes or until the vegetables are soft. Add the tomatoes, wine and cherries, and bring to the boil. Transfer to a large casserole dish.

Heat the remaining oil in the frying pan, add the pork loin and cook for 2 minutes each side or until golden brown. Nestle the pork into the vegetables, then cover the casserole with a lid or foil and cook in the oven for 30 minutes.

Remove the lid and cook for a further 15 minutes. Cut the pork into slices and arrange on shallow serving dishes with the vegetables. Sprinkle with parsley and serve with steamed vegetables.

1 serve = 1½ units protein, 2 units vegetables,
½ unit fruit, 2 units fats

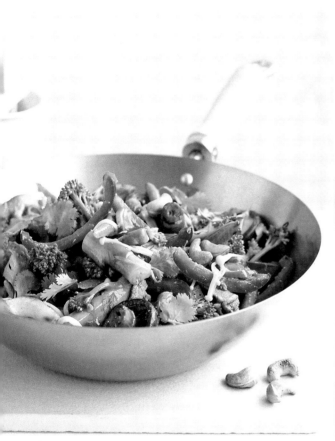

Stir-fried pork with green beans & mixed mushrooms

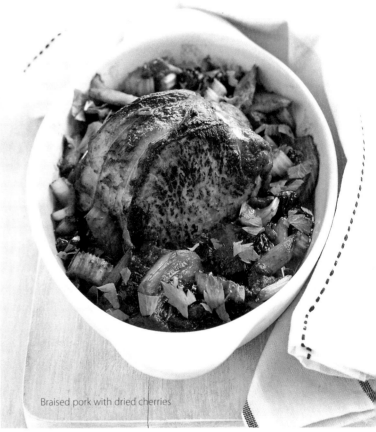

Braised pork with dried cherries

Pork cutlets with cabbage, parsnips & raisins

Dinner Serves 4

4 parsnips, peeled and cut into 5 cm chunks

2 tablespoons canola oil

4 × 150 g pork loin cutlets, trimmed

1 tablespoon sterol spread

1 red onion, finely diced

2 teaspoons caraway seeds

400 g green cabbage, finely shredded

½ cup raisins

½ cup apple juice

1 tablespoon shredded sage leaves

apple sauce

Preheat the oven to 200°C and line a baking tray with baking paper. Place the parsnips on the tray and drizzle with 1 tablespoon of the canola oil. Season with freshly ground black pepper and bake for 20 minutes or until golden brown and tender.

Meanwhile, heat the remaining oil in a heavy-based frying pan over medium heat, add the cutlets and cook for 6 minutes each side or until cooked to your liking. Set aside on a plate and cover with foil.

Return the pan to the heat, add the sterol spread, onion and caraway seeds and cook for 1 minute or until the onion is soft. Add the cabbage, raisins and apple juice and cook for 5 minutes or until the cabbage is soft and the liquid has been absorbed. Stir in the sage.

Divide the parsnips and the cabbage mixture among serving plates, top with the pork and serve with apple sauce.

1 serve = 1½ units protein, 1½ units vegetables,
½ unit fruit, 3 units fats

Thai beef kebabs

Dinner Serves 4

600 g lean rump steak

2 teaspoons canola oil

juice and finely grated zest of 1 lime

1 long green chilli, seeded and finely chopped

1 clove garlic, crushed

2 teaspoons finely chopped ginger

Green chilli sauce

⅓ cup low-fat natural yoghurt

1 long green chilli, seeded and finely chopped

½ cup roughly chopped mint

½ cup roughly chopped coriander

¼ cup roughly chopped Thai basil

If using bamboo skewers, soak them in cold water for 30 minutes before use (you'll need eight).

Cut the beef into 4 cm cubes and thread evenly onto the skewers. Place in a ceramic dish. Whisk together the oil, lime juice and zest, chilli, garlic and ginger in a small bowl and pour over the skewers. Cover with plastic wrap and marinate in the fridge for 20 minutes.

To make the green chilli sauce, place all the sauce ingredients in a food processor and whiz until smooth.

Preheat a chargrill or barbecue to medium. Cook the skewers for 4 minutes each side or until the beef is cooked to your liking, basting with any remaining marinade. Serve with the green chilli sauce and a fresh Sesame Spinach Salad (see page 199).

1 serve = 1½ units protein, ½ unit vegetables

Pork cutlets with cabbage, parsnips & raisins

Thai beef kebabs

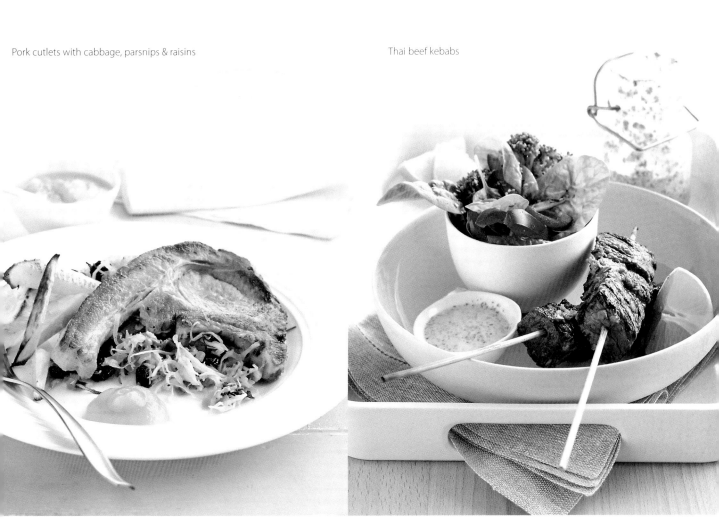

Winter lamb casserole

Dinner Serves 4

- 600 g trimmed lamb shoulder, cut into 4 cm chunks
- 2 tablespoons wholemeal plain flour
- 2 tablespoons canola oil
- 2 onions, diced
- 2 carrots, peeled and sliced
- 3 sticks celery, sliced
- ½ cup red wine
- 1 litre salt-reduced beef stock
- 1 × 400 g tin salt-reduced chopped tomatoes
- 1 tablespoon salt-reduced Worcestershire sauce
- 1 tablespoon chopped rosemary
- ¼ cup roughly chopped flat-leaf parsley
- 1 tablespoon finely grated lemon zest

Preheat the oven to 170°C. Dredge the lamb chunks in the flour and shake off any excess.

Heat 1 tablespoon of the oil in a heavy-based flameproof casserole dish (with a lid) over medium heat. Add the lamb in batches and cook for 4 minutes each side or until golden. Remove from the pan.

Add the remaining oil and cook the onion, carrot and celery for 2 minutes or until the vegetables start to soften. Add the wine, stock, tomatoes, Worcestershire sauce and rosemary and bring to the boil. Return the lamb to the dish.

Cover, transfer to the oven and cook for 40 minutes. Remove the lid and cook for a further 10 minutes. Stir in the parsley and lemon zest and serve with steamed pumpkin and greens.

1 serve = 1½ units protein, 1 unit vegetables, 2 units fats

Oregano & lemon lamb with green beans & butternut pumpkin

Dinner Serves 4

- 500 g butternut pumpkin, peeled and cut into 4 cm chunks
- 2 tablespoons olive oil
- 4 × 150 g lamb backstraps
- 2 teaspoons dried oregano
- juice and finely grated zest of 1 lemon
- 2 cloves garlic, finely chopped
- 150 g green beans, trimmed

Preheat the oven to 200°C and line a roasting tin with baking paper. Place the pumpkin in the tin, drizzle with 1 tablespoon of the olive oil and toss to coat. Roast for 25 minutes or until tender.

Meanwhile, combine the lamb, oregano, lemon juice and zest, garlic and the remaining olive oil in a ceramic dish, then leave to marinate for 10 minutes.

Heat a chargrill pan over medium heat and cook the lamb for 4 minutes each side or until cooked to your liking. Set aside on a plate to rest.

Bring a saucepan of water to the boil, add the beans and cook for 2 minutes until bright green and still crisp.

Slice the lamb on an angle and serve with the beans and roasted pumpkin.

1 serve = 1½ units protein, 2 units vegetables, 2 units fats

Winter lamb casserole

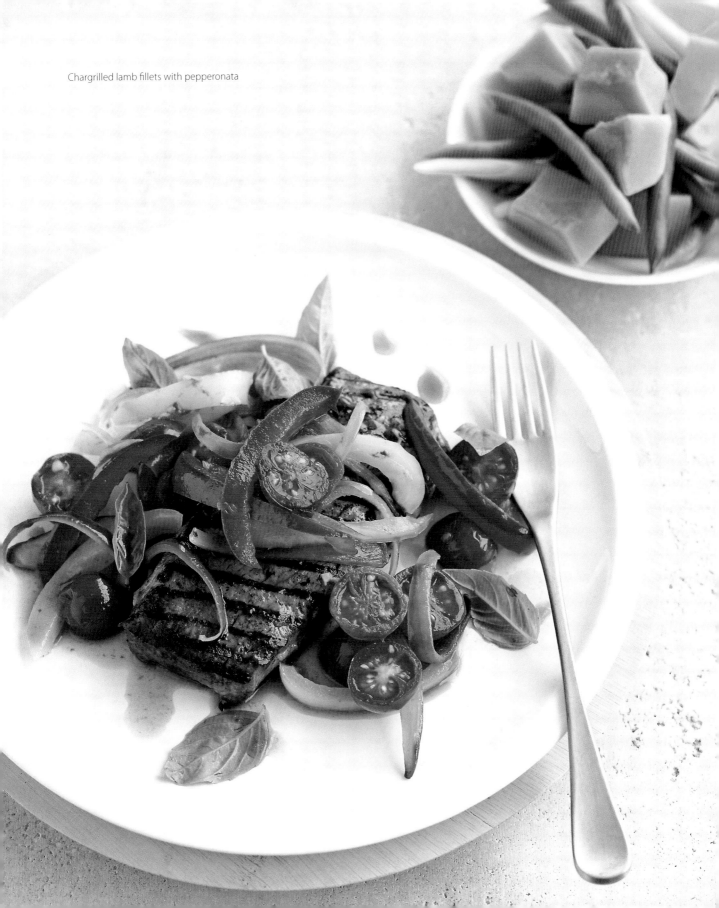

Chargrilled lamb fillets with pepperonata

Chargrilled lamb fillets with pepperonata

Dinner Serves 4

- 600 g lamb fillet, cut into four pieces
- 2 tablespoons olive oil
- 2 red capsicums, sliced
- 1 yellow capsicum, sliced
- 1 red onion, finely sliced
- 2 cloves garlic, finely sliced
- 1 punnet cherry tomatoes, halved
- 1 cup basil leaves

Preheat a chargrill or barbecue to medium–high and cook the lamb fillets for 3 minutes each side or until cooked to your liking. Transfer to a plate, cover with foil and leave to rest for 5 minutes.

To make the pepperonata, heat a large frying pan over medium heat and add the olive oil, capsicum, onion and garlic. Cook for 3 minutes until the capsicum starts to soften. Add the tomatoes and cook for a further 5 minutes until they begin to collapse, then stir in the basil.

Serve the lamb fillets with pepperonata, steamed beans and carrots or pumpkin.

1 serve = 1½ units protein, 1½ units vegetables, 2 units fats

Lamb & spinach meatballs with spicy tomato sauce

Dinner Serves 4

- 500 g lean minced lamb
- 1 tablespoon pine nuts, roughly chopped
- 1 red onion, finely diced
- 2 cloves garlic, crushed
- 2 teaspoons garam masala
- 1 egg, lightly beaten
- 2 tablespoons roughly chopped coriander
- 2 tablespoons roughly chopped mint
- 150 g baby spinach leaves, roughly chopped
- olive oil spray
- 1 tablespoon hot mango chutney
- 700 ml salt-reduced tomato passata (tomato puree)

Preheat the oven to 180°C.

Place the lamb, pine nuts, onion, garlic, garam masala, egg, coriander, mint and spinach in a large bowl. Mix together well, then roll into 12 even meatballs.

Heat a large non-stick frying pan over medium–high heat and spray lightly with olive oil. Cook the meatballs for 5 minutes until evenly brown, then transfer to an ovenproof ceramic dish.

Mix the chutney and tomato passata together and pour over the meatballs. Cover loosely with foil, place in the oven and cook for 20 minutes or until the meatballs are cooked through. Serve with salad.

1 serve = 1½ units protein, 2 units vegetables

SANDWICH SUGGESTIONS

Use wholewheat Mountain Bread to make your lunchtime sandwiches (1 unit carbohydrate only) and you will then have an extra carbohydrate unit to enjoy at dinner. If you are on Option 1, this will mean 1 unit carbohydrate at dinner (rather than none), and if you are on Option 2 you could have 2 units carbohydrate at dinner (instead of 1). Add 1 teaspoon sterol spread to each slice (2 units sterol).

- 40 g smoked trout with 20 g avocado, red onion and 1 cup baby cos lettuce
  1 serve = ½ unit protein, 2 units carbohydrates, 1 unit vegetables, 1 unit fats

- 40 g tuna tinned in spring water with 2 teaspoons fat-free mayonnaise, sliced celery and spring onions and 1 cup butter lettuce
  1 serve = ½ unit protein, 2 units carbohydrates, 1 unit vegetables

- Curried egg (1 egg mashed with 2 teaspoons fat-free mayonnaise, low-salt curry powder and lemon juice) with sliced cucumber and 1 cup watercress
  1 serve = ½ unit protein, 2 units carbohydrates, 1 unit vegetables

- 40 g sliced chicken breast with 1 tablespoon low-fat natural yoghurt, cucumber, dried mint, sliced tomato and 1 cup lettuce
  1 serve = ½ unit protein, 2 units carbohydrates, 1 unit vegetables

- 40 g pink salmon tinned in spring water with low-salt gherkins, lemon juice and 1 cup rocket
  1 serve = ½ unit protein, 2 units carbohydrates 1 unit vegetables

- 40 g turkey with 20 g low-fat ricotta, sliced tomato and 1 cup baby spinach
  1 serve = ½ unit protein, 2 units carbohydrates, ½ unit cheese, 1 unit vegetables

- 40 g turkey with 20 g avocado, 20 g cranberry sauce, sliced tomato and 1 cup baby cos lettuce
  1 serve = ½ unit protein, 1 unit carbohydrates, 1 unit vegetables, 1 unit fats

- 40 g lean roast beef with grated fresh horseradish (or salt-reduced prepared horseradish) mixed with 2 teaspoons fat-free mayonnaise, sliced tomato, grated carrot and 1 cup watercress
  1 serve = ½ unit protein, 2 units carbohydrates, 1 unit vegetables, 1 unit fats

SALAD SUGGESTIONS

- **Beetroot and asparagus salad**
  Tinned baby beets, mesclun salad (mixed baby leaves), finely sliced fennel and blanched asparagus spears. Drizzle with fat-free balsamic dressing.

- **Tomato and herb salad**
  Vine-ripened tomatoes, finely sliced red onion, torn basil and mint leaves and rocket. Drizzle with olive oil (count fat units) and balsamic vinegar.

- **Green vegie salad**
  Blanched and refreshed broccoli florets, trimmed snow peas, Lebanese cucumber, witlof, parsley and mint leaves. Drizzle with fat-free ranch dressing.

- **Pumpkin salad**
  Roasted butternut pumpkin, finely sliced spring onions (scallions), low-fat feta and halved cherry tomatoes. Drizzle with fat-free balsamic dressing.

- **Sesame spinach salad**
  Baby spinach leaves, sesame seeds, blanched and refreshed broccolini and finely sliced red capsicum. Drizzle with low-salt soy sauce, sesame oil (count fats units) and rice-wine vinegar.

VEGETABLE SUGGESTIONS

- Sliced zucchini, button squash and broccoli cooked with crushed garlic, olive oil and parsley

- Steamed or boiled carrots and green beans with roasted red onion and fat-free honey soy dressing

- Steamed corn cob, snow peas and sweet potato, drizzled with olive oil and balsamic vinegar

- Roasted tomatoes and leek with balsamic vinegar and shredded basil

- Frozen spinach gently heated through with a knob of sterol spread, finely grated lemon zest and a sprinkle of grated parmesan

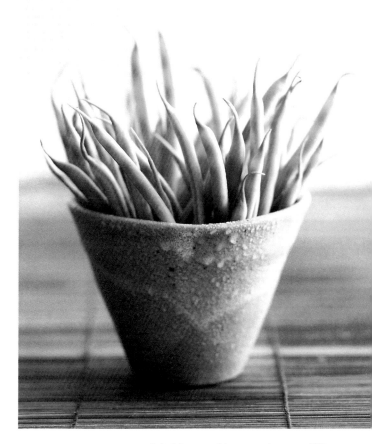

Barbecue for 6

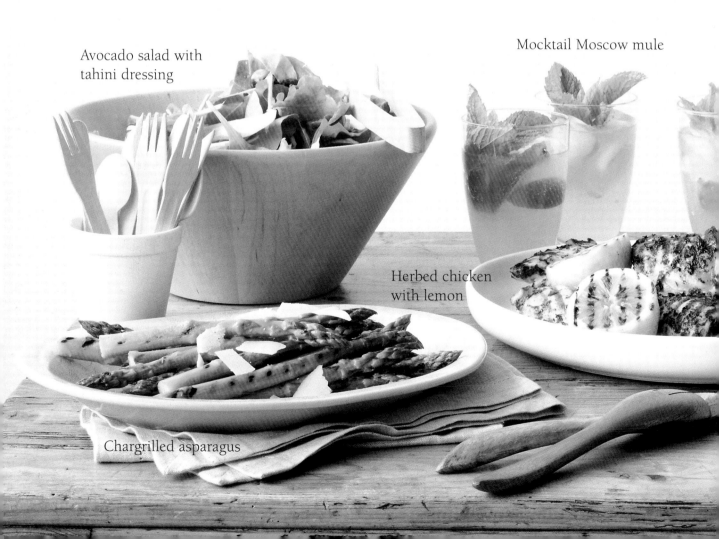

Avocado salad with
tahini dressing

Mocktail Moscow mule

Herbed chicken
with lemon

Chargrilled asparagus

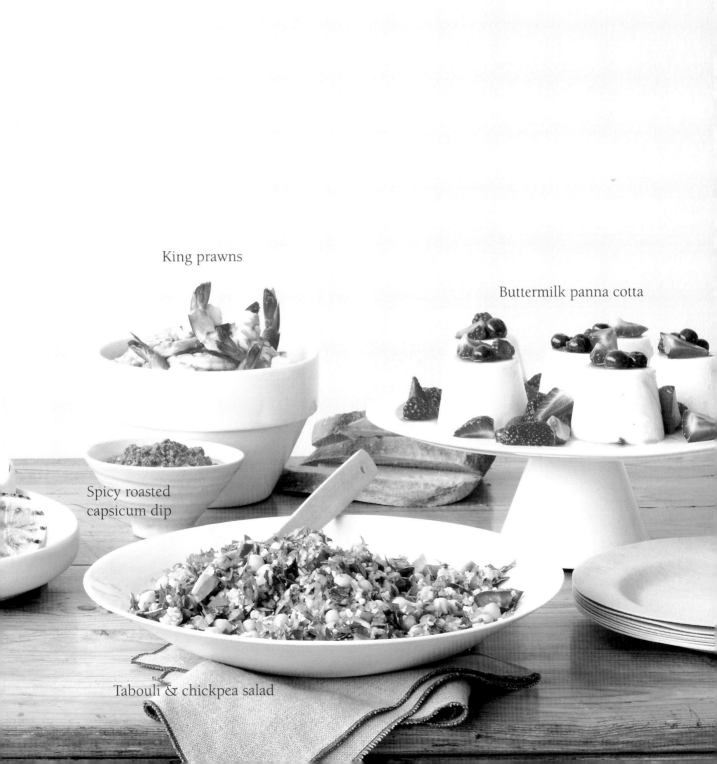

King prawns

Buttermilk panna cotta

Spicy roasted
capsicum dip

Tabouli & chickpea salad

Mocktail Moscow mule

Free

> ice cubes
> Angostura bitters
> 6 sprigs mint
> ½ lime, cut into 6 wedges
> low-joule ginger beer

Fill six highball glasses with ice. Splash a couple of drops of bitters into each glass, and add a sprig of mint and a lime wedge, squeezed. Fill each glass with ginger beer.

Herbed chicken with lemon

> 2 cups roughly torn coriander
> 1 cup roughly torn basil
> 1 cup roughly torn mint
> 2 cloves garlic, roughly chopped
> 1 tablespoon olive oil
> ¼ cup lemon juice
> 1 teaspoon ground cardamom
> 6 skinless chicken thigh cutlets (with bone),
>   skin removed
> 3 lemons, halved

Place the herbs, garlic, oil, lemon juice and cardamom in a food processor and whiz until combined. Transfer to a large bowl.

Cut three slashes into each chicken thigh, then place in the bowl with the herb paste. Rub in well, cover with plastic wrap and place in the fridge for 30 minutes to marinate.

Preheat a barbecue plate to high. Cook the chicken for 8 minutes each side or until cooked through. Remove and set aside. Cook the lemon halves, cut-side down, for 3 minutes or until golden and juicy, and serve with the chicken.

1 serve = 1 unit protein

King prawns with crusty bread

> 1 kg cooked king prawns, peeled and deveined,
>   tails intact
> 2 lemons, cut into wedges
> 6 slices crusty sourdough bread
> Spicy Roasted Capsicum Dip (see page 172)

Place the prawns in a large serving bowl. Serve with lemon wedges, slices of sourdough and a bowl of Spicy Roasted Capsicum Dip.

1 serve = 1 unit protein, 1 unit carbohydrates

Chargrilled asparagus

Free

> 3 bunches green asparagus, trimmed
> olive oil spray
> 1 tablespoon olive oil
> 2 tablespoons lemon juice
> 1 tablespoon grated parmesan

Heat a barbecue plate to high. Lightly spray the asparagus spears with olive oil and cook for 2 minutes each side (they will be bright green and lightly charred). Arrange on a plate.

Combine the olive oil and lemon juice in a bowl. Drizzle the dressing over the asparagus, sprinkle with parmesan and season with freshly ground black pepper. Serve warm.

Tabouli & chickpea salad

½ cup burghul (cracked wheat)

2 teaspoons finely grated lemon zest

2 tablespoons lemon juice

2 tomatoes, diced

1 × 400 g tin salt-reduced chickpeas,
    drained and rinsed

3 cups roughly chopped flat-leaf parsley

2 cups roughly chopped mint

Place the burghul in a heatproof dish and pour over 1 cup boiling water. Cover and leave for 10 minutes, then drain well, squeezing out any excess moisture with your hands. Add the remaining ingredients and mix well.

1 serve = 1 unit carbohydrates

Avocado salad with tahini dressing

50 g baby rocket

2 witlof, leaves separated

50 g baby spinach leaves

1 avocado, peeled and sliced

⅓ cup pitted kalamata olives

Tahini dressing

2 teaspoons tahini

1 tablespoon lemon juice

1 clove garlic, crushed

2 tablespoons olive oil

To make the dressing, place all the dressing ingredients and 1 tablespoon boiling water in a screw-top jar and shake until smooth and well combined.

Place the rocket, witlof and baby spinach in a serving dish and mix well. Scatter the avocado and olives over the salad and drizzle with the tahini dressing.

1 serve = 2 units fats

Buttermilk panna cotta

2 cups buttermilk

2 tablespoons caster sugar, plus 2 teaspoons, extra

1 vanilla bean, split

1½ tablespoons powdered gelatine

300 ml low-fat vanilla sterol yoghurt

300 g mixed berries

¼ cup Crème de Cassis

Place the buttermilk, sugar and vanilla bean in a small saucepan and stir over low heat until the sugar dissolves.

Pour ¼ cup boiling water into a small jug, sprinkle in the gelatine and whisk until it dissolves. Pour into the buttermilk mixture and stir. Strain and discard the vanilla bean.

Place the yoghurt in a bowl and fold in the gelatine mixture. Pour into 6 × 125 ml dariole moulds, then cover and place in the fridge for 3 hours or until set.

Combine the berries, extra sugar and Crème de Cassis in a bowl, then cover with plastic wrap and set aside until needed. Serve the panna cotta with the berries in syrup.

1 serve = 2 units indulgence

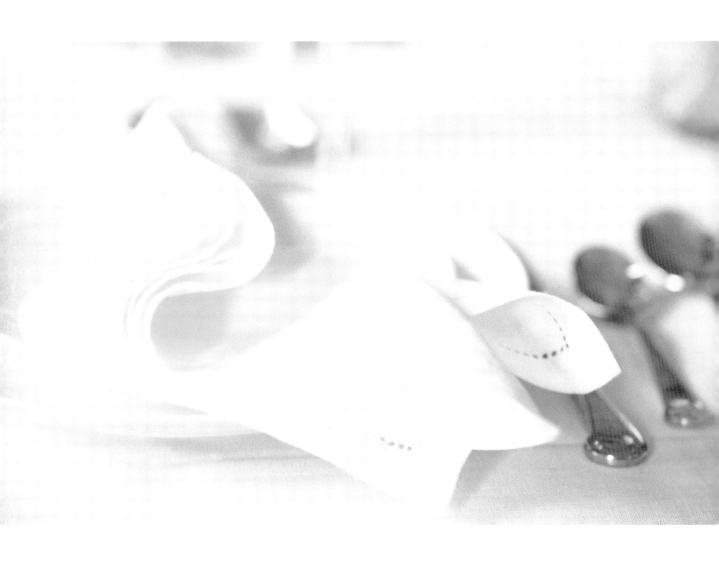

Dinners

Option 2

Tomato & oregano cannelloni

Dinner Serves 4

1 tablespoon olive oil

1 brown onion, finely diced

2 sticks celery, finely diced

1 clove garlic, crushed

400 g Sanitarium Vegie Delights Mince

1 cup salt-reduced vegetable stock

¼ cup red wine

1 tablespoon salt-reduced tomato paste

2 tomatoes, finely diced

1½ teaspoons dried oregano

2 tablespoons chopped flat-leaf parsley

olive oil spray

375 g fresh lasagne sheets

2 cups salt-reduced tomato passata (tomato puree)

½ cup low-fat ricotta

2 tablespoons low-fat sterol milk

¼ cup low-fat pizza cheese

Heat the oil in a frying pan over medium heat and cook the onion, celery and garlic for 5 minutes or until softened. Add the Vegie Mince, stock, red wine and tomato paste and cook for 8 minutes. Stir in the tomato, oregano and parsley, then reduce the heat and simmer for 15 minutes. Set aside to cool slightly. Preheat the oven to 200°C and spray a large ceramic baking dish with olive oil.

Cut the lasagne sheets in half crossways. Place ⅓ cup of the filling along one side of each sheet and roll up to enclose the filling. Transfer to the prepared dish and spoon the tomato passata over the top.

In a small bowl, mix together the ricotta and milk. Spoon this mixture over the passata, scatter with the cheese and bake for 35–40 minutes or until golden. Serve with salad.

1 serve = 1 unit protein, 1 unit carbohydrates,
½ unit cheese, 1½ units vegetables

Baked beans

Dinner Serves 4

2 tablespoons olive oil

1 red onion, finely chopped

1 clove garlic, crushed

1 × 400 g tin salt-reduced chopped tomatoes

2 teaspoons brown sugar

Tabasco sauce, to taste

1 × 400 g tin salt-reduced cannellini beans, drained and rinsed

¼ cup roughly chopped flat-leaf parsley

4 slices wholegrain toast

Heat the oil in a large heavy-based saucepan over medium heat and cook the onion and garlic for 2–3 minutes or until softened. Add the chopped tomato, brown sugar and Tabasco sauce. Bring to the boil, then reduce the heat and add the beans. Cover and simmer for 15 minutes or until the sauce is thick. Stir in the parsley and serve with wholegrain toast and a green salad.

1 serve = 1 unit protein, 1 unit carbohydrates, 1 unit fats

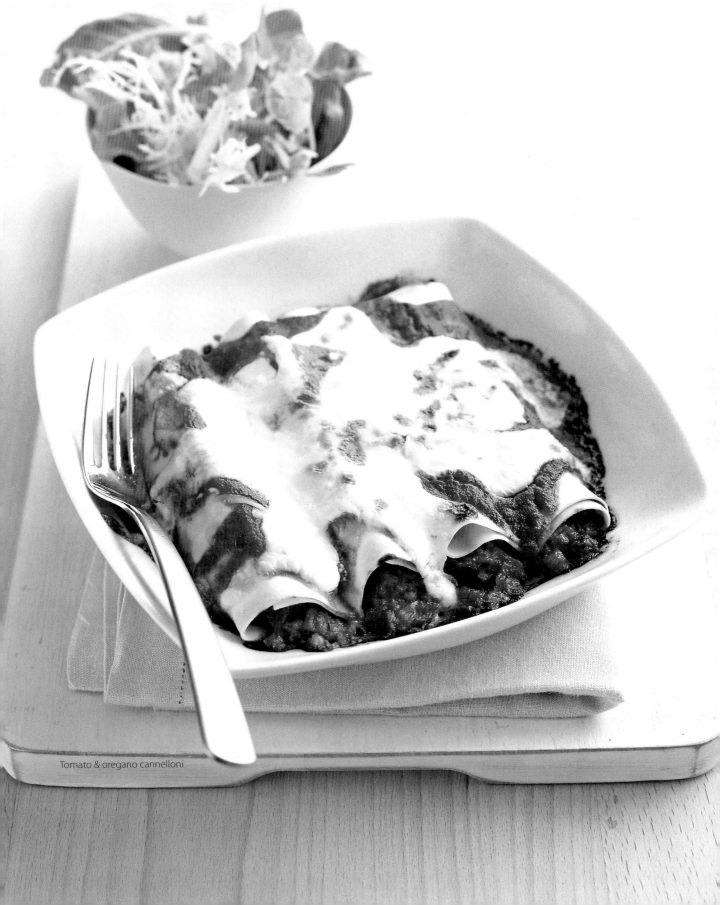

Tomato & oregano cannelloni

Curried sweet potato cakes

Dinner Serves 4

- 500 g sweet potato, peeled and cut into 3 cm chunks
- 1 tablespoon sterol spread
- 1 large onion, finely diced
- 1 clove garlic, crushed
- 1 tablespoon low-salt curry powder
- 1 × 400 g tin salt-reduced lentils, drained and rinsed
- 1 cup frozen peas, thawed
- ¼ cup roughly chopped coriander
- 1 cup fresh wholemeal breadcrumbs (made from day-old wholegrain bread)
- 1 tablespoon canola oil
- 2 limes, halved

Place the sweet potato in a saucepan of water, bring to the boil and cook for 10 minutes or until tender. Drain well and mash with a potato masher. Allow to cool slightly.

Heat the sterol spread in a frying pan over medium heat and cook the onion and garlic for 2 minutes or until softened. Add the curry powder and cook for a further minute. Remove from the heat and combine in a bowl with the sweet potato, lentils, peas and coriander. Form the mixture into eight patties. Place the breadcrumbs on a shallow plate. Coat the patties in the breadcrumbs, shaking off any excess.

Heat the oil in a large non-stick frying pan over medium heat. Cook the patties for 5 minutes each side or until golden and heated through. Remove and keep warm.

Return the pan to the heat and add the lime halves, cut-side down. Cook for 3 minutes or until golden and juicy.

Serve the potato cakes and charred limes with steamed green beans or salad and sweet chilli sauce on the side.

1 serve = 1 unit protein, 1 unit carbohydrates, 1 unit vegetables, 2 units fats

Vegetable samosa parcels

Dinner Serves 4

- 500 g pumpkin, peeled and cut into 1 cm cubes
- canola oil spray
- 1 tablespoon canola oil
- 1 onion, finely diced
- 2 teaspoons grated ginger
- 1 clove garlic, crushed
- 400 g Sanitarium Vegie Delights Mince
- 1 teaspoon ground cumin
- 1 tablespoon low-salt curry powder
- 1 tomato, finely diced
- 1 cup frozen peas
- ¼ cup roughly chopped coriander
- 1 tablespoon finely grated lemon zest
- 8 sheets filo pastry
- 1 tablespoon sesame seeds

Preheat the oven to 180°C. Place the pumpkin on a baking tray, lightly spray with oil and bake for 20 minutes. Set aside.

Heat the oil in a large frying pan over medium heat and cook the onion, ginger and garlic for 2 minutes. Add the Vegie Mince and spices and cook for 5 minutes. Add the pumpkin and tomato and mix. Stir in the peas, coriander and lemon zest, then remove from heat and leave to cool.

Lay out one sheet of filo on a clean surface and spray with oil. Place the next sheet on top and spray with oil. Repeat to make two stacks of four sheets, then cut the stacks in half to make four rectangles. Line a baking tray with baking paper. Spoon the mixture onto the pastry along the short edge. Fold the sides in and roll up into triangular parcels. Place the parcels on the baking tray, seam-side down. Spray the top with oil, sprinkle with sesame seeds and bake for 20 minutes. Serve with mango chutney, raita and a salad.

1 serve = 1 unit protein, 1 unit carbohydrates, 1 unit vegetables, 1 unit fats

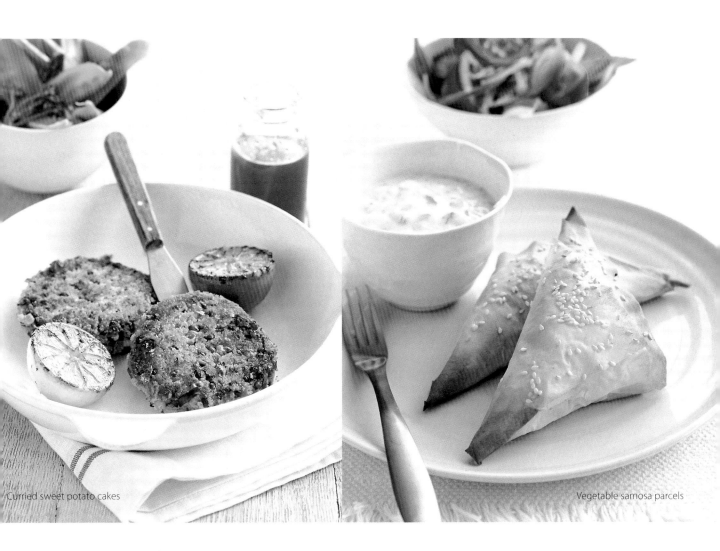

Curried sweet potato cakes

Vegetable samosa parcels

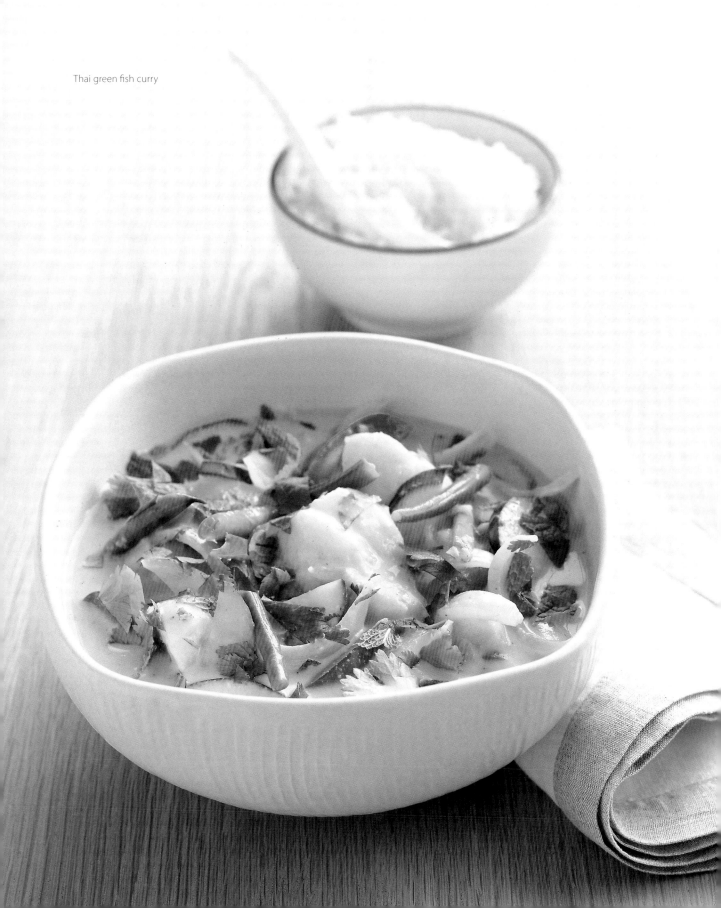

Thai green fish curry

Thai green fish curry

Dinner Serves 4

olive or canola oil spray

1 brown onion, cut into thin wedges

2 cloves garlic, crushed

1 × 3 cm piece ginger, finely grated

2 tablespoons green curry paste

400 ml light coconut milk

½ cup salt-reduced chicken stock

2 zucchini, thinly sliced

1 red capsicum, cut into thin strips

50 g green beans, trimmed and cut
into 3 cm lengths

2 tablespoons low-salt soy sauce

juice of 2 limes

1 tablespoon brown sugar

400 g white fish fillets (barramundi, gemfish
or flathead), cut into 5 cm chunks

½ cup roughly chopped coriander

½ cup roughly torn mint

320 g steamed long-grain rice

Heat a large non-stick frying pan over medium heat, spray with oil and cook the onion, garlic and ginger for 2 minutes. Stir in the curry paste and cook for a further minute or until aromatic. Add the coconut milk and stock and bring to the boil, then reduce the heat and simmer for 5 minutes. Add the zucchini, capsicum and beans.

Combine the soy sauce, half the lime juice and sugar in a small bowl, then stir into the curry. Add the fish and simmer for 1 minute or until cooked through. Stir in half the herbs.

Spoon the curry into serving dishes, top with the remaining herbs, squeeze over the remaining lime juice and serve with steamed rice.

1 serve = 1 unit protein, 1 unit carbohydrates,
½ unit dairy, 1½ units vegetables

Chargrilled salmon with lentils, spinach & yoghurt

Dinner Serves 4

1 tablespoon olive oil

1 red onion, finely sliced

1 clove garlic, finely sliced

4 Roma tomatoes, diced

1 × 400 g tin salt-reduced lentils, drained
and rinsed

150 g green beans, trimmed and cut into
5 cm lengths

100 g baby spinach leaves

1 tablespoon finely grated lemon zest

2 tablespoons low-fat natural yoghurt mixed
with 1 tablespoon water

¼ cup roughly chopped flat-leaf parsley

4 × 100 g salmon fillets

canola oil spray

lemon wedges

Heat the oil in a large non-stick frying pan over medium heat and cook the onion and garlic for 1 minute or until the onion begins to soften. Add the tomato, lentils, beans and spinach and cook until the spinach starts to wilt. Stir in the lemon zest, yoghurt and parsley and remove from heat.

Heat a chargrill or barbecue to high. Lightly spray the salmon fillets with canola oil and cook for 2 minutes each side or until cooked to your liking.

Spoon the lentils into shallow serving dishes, top with the salmon and serve with lemon wedges.

1 serve = 1 unit protein, 1 unit carbohydrates,
1½ units vegetables, 1 unit fats

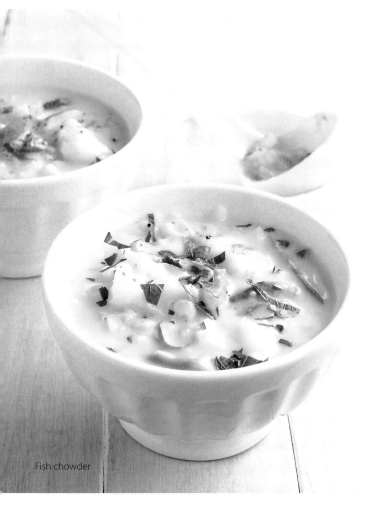

Fish chowder

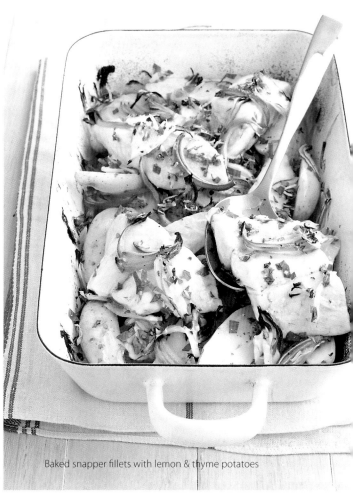

Baked snapper fillets with lemon & thyme potatoes

Fish chowder

Dinner Serves 4

1 tablespoon olive oil

1 onion, finely chopped

2 sticks celery, finely chopped

1 clove garlic, crushed

1 tablespoon wholemeal plain flour

1 cup low-fat sterol milk

3 cups salt-reduced chicken stock

2 corn cobs, kernels removed

400 g desiree potatoes, peeled and cut
   into 1 cm cubes

400 g white fish fillets (perch, gemfish, cod
   or flathead), cut into 2 cm chunks

100 g green beans, trimmed and cut into
   1 cm lengths

150 ml evaporated milk

¼ cup roughly chopped flat-leaf parsley

Heat the oil in a large heavy-based saucepan over medium heat and cook the onion, celery and garlic for 2 minutes or until soft.

Add the flour and cook for 1 minute, stirring constantly. Slowly stir in the milk and then the stock, corn and potato. Bring to the boil, then reduce the heat and simmer for 5 minutes or until the potato is tender. Lightly crush the potato with a masher, to thicken the chowder.

Add the fish and beans and simmer for 5 minutes or until the fish is just cooked and opaque. Stir in the evaporated milk and parsley and season with freshly ground black pepper. Spoon into serving bowls.

1 serve = 1 unit protein, 1 unit carbohydrates,
½ unit dairy, 1½ units vegetables, 1 unit fats

Baked snapper fillets with lemon & thyme potatoes

Dinner Serves 4

600 g kipfler potatoes, scrubbed and
   halved lengthways

1 bulb fennel, finely sliced

1 clove garlic

1 red onion, finely sliced

juice and finely grated zest of 1 lemon

2 teaspoons finely chopped thyme

½ cup white wine or salt-reduced chicken stock

2 teaspoons olive oil

4 × 100 g snapper fillets, skin on, cut in half
   crossways on an angle

Preheat the oven to 200°C and line a baking dish with baking paper. Place the potatoes in a medium-sized saucepan, cover with cold water and place over medium heat. Bring to the boil, then simmer for 10 minutes or until the potatoes are just tender. Drain, then place in the baking tray, along with the fennel, garlic and onion. Mix the lemon juice and zest, thyme, wine or stock and olive oil in a small jug and pour over the potato mixture. Bake for 30 minutes.

Remove the dish from the oven and sit the snapper pieces on the vegetables. Return to the oven and cook for a further 10 minutes or until the fish is cooked through.

Serve with a crisp salad.

1 serve = 1 unit protein, 1 unit carbohydrates,
1 unit vegetables

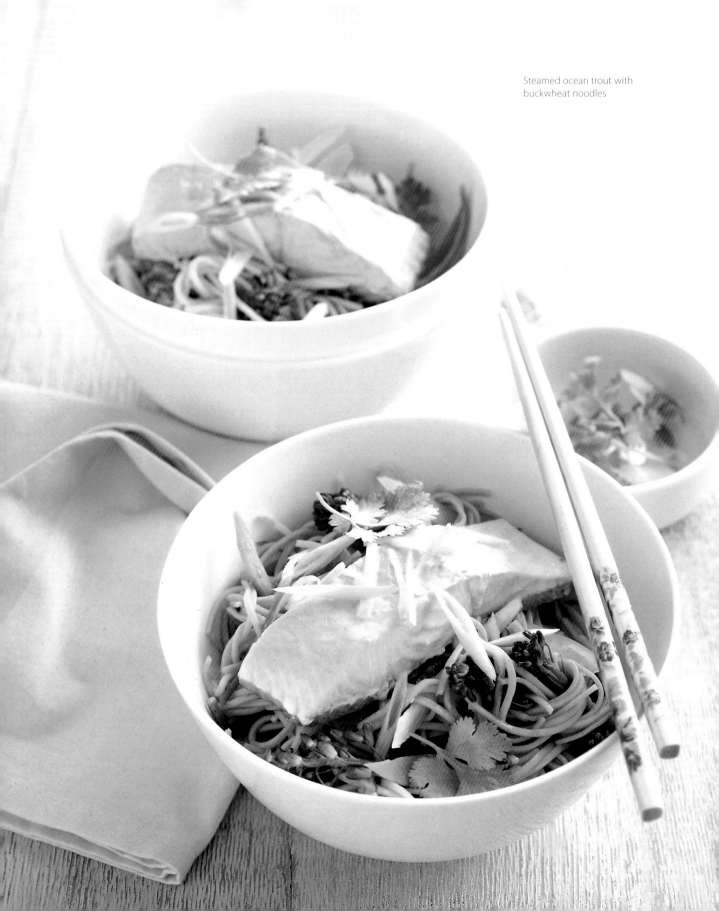

Steamed ocean trout with
buckwheat noodles

Steamed ocean trout with buckwheat noodles

Dinner Serves 4

- 4 × 100 g ocean trout fillets
- 2 tablespoons Chinese rice wine or dry sherry
- 1 × 3 cm piece ginger, finely shredded
- ½ cup coriander leaves
- 4 spring onions (scallions), finely sliced on an angle
- lime wedges

Buckwheat noodles

- juice of 1 lime
- 2 tablespoons salt-reduced tamari
- 1 teaspoon sesame oil
- 320 g buckwheat noodles
- 200 g snow peas, trimmed
- 1 bunch broccolini, cut into small florets
- 1 zucchini, thickly sliced
- 1 yellow capsicum, sliced

Preheat the oven to 200°C. Place the trout, skin-side down, in a ceramic dish. Pour the rice wine and ¼ cup water over the fish, then sprinkle with the ginger. Cover tightly with foil and cook in the oven for 5–10 minutes or until cooked to your liking.

Meanwhile, prepare the noodles. Whisk together the lime juice, tamari and sesame oil in a small bowl. Cook the noodles according to the packet instructions, adding the snow peas, broccoli and zucchini 1 minute before the end of the cooking time. Drain and toss with the dressing and capsicum.

Divide the noodles and vegetables among serving plates and top with the ocean trout. Scatter with coriander and spring onion and serve with lime wedges.

1 serve = 1 unit protein, 1 unit carbohydrates, 2 units vegetables

Tuna pasta bake

Dinner Serves 4

- 300 g fusilli pasta
- 2 tablespoons sterol spread
- 1 onion, finely chopped
- 2 tablespoons plain flour
- 2½ cups low-fat sterol milk, warmed
- 1 × 425 g tin tuna in spring water, drained and flaked
- 2 tablespoons lemon juice
- ½ cup frozen peas
- 160 g low-fat cheddar, grated
- ¼ cup finely chopped flat-leaf parsley
- 2 teaspoons finely grated lemon zest
- ½ cup fresh wholegrain breadcrumbs (made from day-old wholegrain bread)

Preheat the oven to 200°C.

Cook the fusilli according to the packet instructions. Drain well and refresh under cold running water. Set aside in a large bowl.

Meanwhile, melt the sterol spread in a saucepan over medium heat and cook the onion for 2 minutes or until soft. Add the flour and stir to coat the onion, then gradually add the milk to make a smooth sauce. Simmer for 2 minutes, stirring constantly.

Pour the sauce over the pasta. Add the tuna, lemon juice, peas and half the cheese and mix well. Spoon the tuna pasta into a ceramic baking dish.

In a small bowl mix together the parsley, lemon zest, breadcrumbs and the remaining cheese. Sprinkle over the pasta and bake for 20 minutes or until golden brown. Serve with a green salad.

1 serve = 1 unit protein, 1 unit carbohydrates, ½ unit dairy, 1 unit cheese, ½ unit vegetables, 2 units fats

Dukkah-crusted salmon with couscous

Dinner Serves 4

4 × 100 g salmon fillets,
   skin removed
1–2 tablespoons dukkah
olive oil spray
lemon wedges

Couscous

⅔ cup instant couscous
1½ teaspoons olive oil
1 tablespoon finely grated
   lemon zest
1½ tablespoons lemon juice
½ cup roughly chopped mint
½ cup roughly chopped basil
4 spring onions (scallions),
   finely sliced

Lemon yoghurt dressing

½ cup low-fat natural yoghurt
2 tablespoons finely shredded mint
1 teaspoon ground cumin
1 teaspoon finely grated lemon zest
2 tablespoons lemon juice

Place the salmon fillets on a plate and press dukkah into both sides.

Place the couscous in a heatproof bowl and pour on the olive oil and ⅔ cup boiling water. Cover with plastic wrap and set aside for 5 minutes or until the liquid has been absorbed. Fluff up the couscous with a fork and stir in the lemon zest, juice, mint, basil and spring onion.

To make the yoghurt dressing, combine all the dressing ingredients in a bowl.

Spray a non-stick frying pan with olive oil and place over medium heat. Cook the salmon for 3 minutes each side or until cooked to your liking.

Divide the couscous among serving plates, top with the salmon and drizzle with the yoghurt dressing. Serve with lemon wedges and steamed vegetables.

1 serve = 1 unit protein, 1 unit carbohydrates

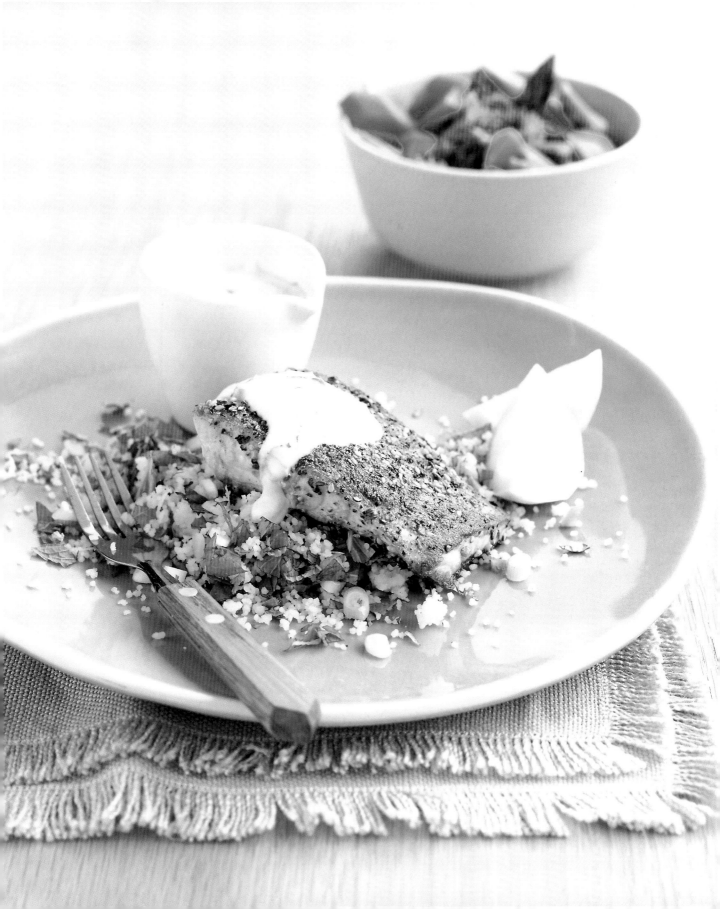

Prawn & salmon risotto with lemon & zucchini

Dinner Serves 4

3 cups salt-reduced chicken stock

2 tablespoons olive oil

1 onion, finely diced

2 cloves garlic, crushed

⅔ cup arborio rice

½ cup white wine

1 zucchini, diced

200 g uncooked prawns, peeled
   and deveined, tails intact

200 g diced salmon fillet

juice and finely grated zest of 1 lemon

½ cup roughly chopped flat-leaf parsley

Bring the stock to the boil in a medium-sized saucepan. Turn off the heat and leave while making the risotto base.

Heat the oil in a large heavy-based saucepan over medium heat and cook the onion and garlic for 2 minutes or until soft. Add the rice and cook, stirring, for 2 minutes until well coated in the oil and onion mixture. Pour in the wine, add the zucchini and simmer until the liquid is absorbed. Stirring constantly, add the stock in batches, ensuring the liquid had been absorbed before adding more. The rice should be tender and moist – if necessary, add a little water.

Add the prawns and salmon and cook, covered, for 2 minutes or until they are cooked through. Stir in the lemon juice and zest and parsley and season well with freshly ground black pepper. Serve immediately with crisp salad leaves.

1 serve = 1 unit protein, 1 unit carbohydrates,
½ unit vegetables, 2 units fats

Linguine with crab, lime & coriander

Dinner Serves 4

120 g dried linguine

2 tablespoons olive oil

1 long red chilli, seeded and finely chopped

400 g cooked crabmeat, picked

1 cup roughly chopped coriander

juice and finely grated zest of 1 lime

2 tomatoes, finely diced

Cook the pasta according to the packet instructions.

Combine the olive oil, chilli, crab, coriander, lime juice, zest and tomato in a large bowl. Add the hot pasta and toss well. Serve immediately with a fresh green salad.

1 serve = 1 unit protein, 1 unit carbohydrates,
½ unit vegetables, 2 units fats

Note: Cooked crabmeat is available in the chilled seafood section of most supermarkets.

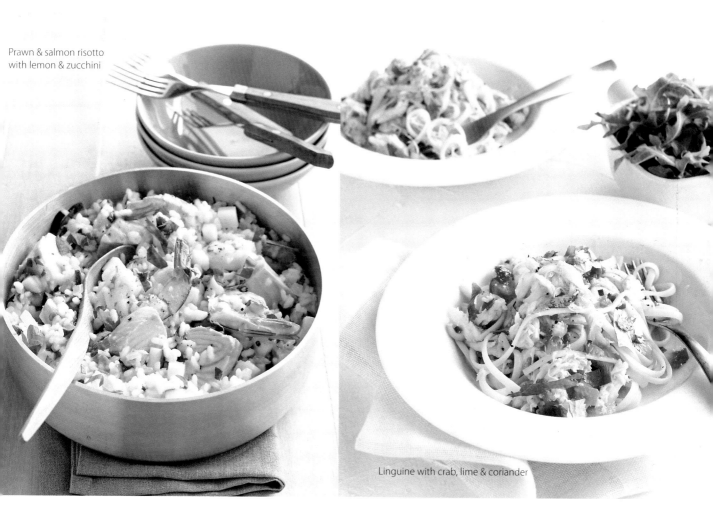

Prawn & salmon risotto
with lemon & zucchini

Linguine with crab, lime & coriander

Smoked chicken, green bean & lentil salad with sesame seeds

Dinner Serves 4

200 g green beans, trimmed
4 marinated artichokes, drained and quartered
400 g smoked chicken breast, sliced
1 × 400 g tin salt-reduced lentils, drained and rinsed
1 witlof, leaves separated
50 g baby rocket
2 tablespoons fat-free balsamic dressing
1 tablespoon sesame seeds, lightly toasted

Blanch the beans in boiling water for 30 seconds until bright green. Drain and refresh in iced water.

Place the artichokes, chicken, lentils, witlof, rocket and dressing in a large bowl and gently toss to combine. Stir in the beans, sprinkle with the sesame seeds and serve immediately.

1 serve = 1 unit protein, 1 unit carbohydrates,
1½ units vegetables

Chicken & vegetable paella

Dinner Serves 4

olive oil spray
400 g chicken thigh fillets, trimmed
    and cut in half crossways
1 large red onion, sliced
1 red capsicum, cut into 2 cm pieces
2 cloves garlic, crushed
120 g arborio rice
1 × 400 g tin salt-reduced chopped tomatoes
1 teaspoon smoked paprika
pinch saffron threads
1 litre salt-reduced chicken stock
150 g green beans, trimmed and cut into
    2 cm pieces
150 g broccoli florets
2 zucchini, finely sliced
1 cup frozen peas
roughly chopped flat-leaf parsley
lemon wedges

Heat a large non-stick frying pan or paella pan over medium heat. Spray with olive oil, then add the chicken and cook for 5 minutes or until golden on both sides. Remove and set aside.

Add the onion, capsicum and garlic to the pan and cook for 3 minutes or until soft. Add the rice, tomato, paprika and saffron, stir to combine, then pour in the stock. Bring to the boil, then reduce the heat to low, cover with a piece of foil and cook for 15 minutes without stirring.

Add the chicken, beans, broccoli, zucchini and peas and cook, uncovered, for a further 10 minutes or until the liquid has been absorbed. Sprinkle the paella with parsley and serve from the pan with lemon wedges.

1 serve = 1 unit protein, 1 unit carbohydrates,
2 units vegetables

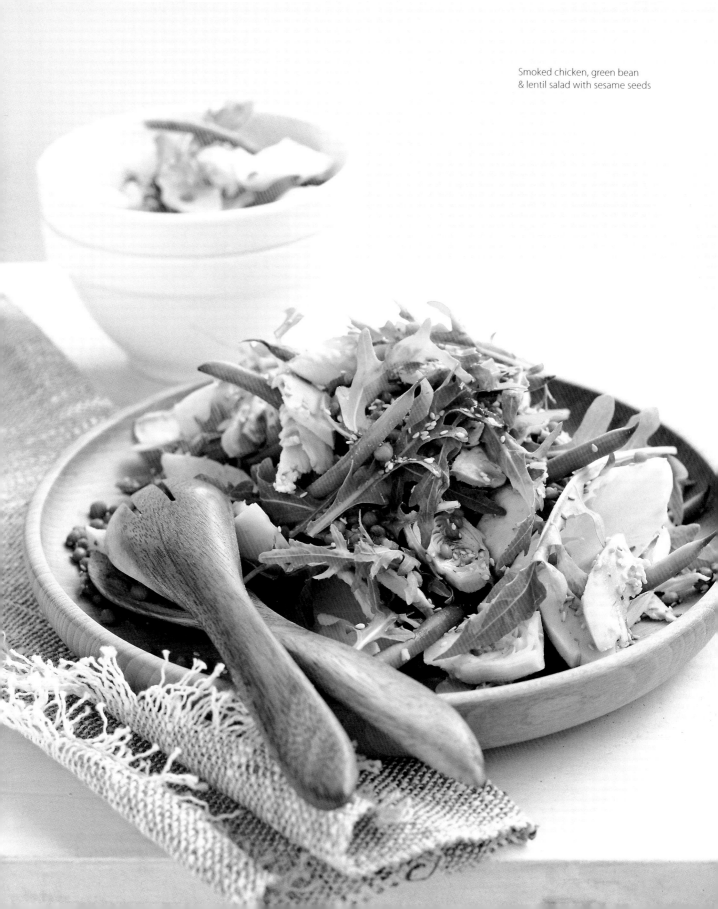

Smoked chicken, green bean & lentil salad with sesame seeds

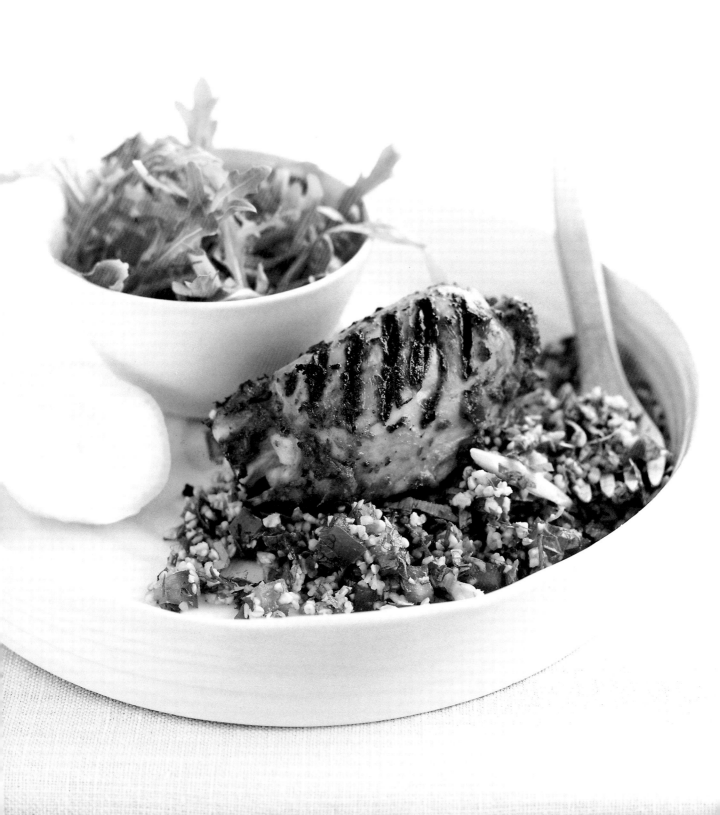

Harissa chicken with tabouli

Dinner Serves 4

750 g skinless chicken thigh cutlets
  (with bone)
lemon wedges

Harissa paste

⅓ cup roughly chopped coriander
1 teaspoon ground cumin
1 teaspoon ground coriander
2 long red chillies, seeded and
  finely chopped
2 cloves garlic, roughly chopped
1 tablespoon olive oil
3 roasted red capsicums, roughly
  chopped (buy in jars)

Tabouli

1 cup burghul (cracked wheat)
juice of 2 lemons
1 teaspoon ground cumin
2 tablespoons extra virgin olive oil
1 bunch flat-leaf parsley, finely
  chopped
½ bunch mint, finely chopped
¼ cup finely chopped coriander
5 spring onions (scallions),
  finely sliced
3 ripe tomatoes, finely diced

To make the harissa paste, place all the paste ingredients in a food processor and whiz until smooth.

Using a sharp knife, cut four shallow incisions into each piece of chicken and place in a bowl. Rub 3 tablespoons of the harissa into the chicken, then cover with plastic wrap and refrigerate for 30 minutes. The remaining harissa will keep for up to 3 weeks if refrigerated in an airtight jar.

To make the tabouli, place the burghul in a bowl and cover with 2 cups boiling water. Leave to absorb for 20 minutes, then drain well, squeezing out any excess water with your hands. Add the lemon juice, cumin, olive oil, parsley, mint, coriander, spring onion and tomato. Season with freshly ground black pepper and mix well.

Heat a chargrill or barbecue to medium. Cook the chicken for 10 minutes each side or until cooked through. Serve with the tabouli and lemon wedges, and a rocket salad if liked.

1 serve = 1 unit protein, 1 unit carbohydrates, 2 units vegetables, 3 units fats

Sesame chicken with soba noodles & plum sauce

Dinner Serves 4

1 egg white, lightly beaten
400 g chicken tenderloins, halved crossways
1 tablespoon sesame seeds
½ long red chilli, seeded and finely sliced
¼ cup plum sauce
1 teaspoon finely chopped ginger
1 teaspoon sesame oil
1 tablespoon rice-wine vinegar
320 g soba noodles
100 g snow peas, trimmed, halved lengthways
   and sliced
1 Lebanese cucumber, sliced
50 g baby spinach leaves
8 spring onions (scallions), sliced on an angle
⅓ cup roughly chopped coriander
1 red capsicum, seeded and finely sliced

Preheat the oven to 200°C and line a baking tray with baking paper. Place the egg white in a bowl, add the chicken and toss to coat. Transfer to the baking tray and sprinkle with sesame seeds. Bake for 10–12 minutes or until the chicken is cooked through.

Meanwhile, combine the chilli, plum sauce, ginger, sesame oil and vinegar in a microwave-safe jug or bowl and cook on high for 30 seconds. Remove and stir well.

Cook the soba noodles according to the packet instructions, adding the snow peas 30 seconds before the end of the cooking time. Drain and toss with half the sauce. Add the chicken and all the remaining ingredients and toss to combine. Divide among serving dishes and drizzle with the remaining sauce.

1 serve = 1 unit protein, 1 unit carbohydrates,
1 unit vegetables

Tuna, corn & coriander patties

Dinner Serves 4

¾ cup short-grain rice (makes approx
   1⅓ cups cooked rice)
1 × 425 g tin tuna in spring water, drained
1 × 125 g tin salt-reduced corn kernels, drained
¼ cup roughly chopped coriander
2 egg whites
1 tablespoon lime juice
4 spring onions (scallions), finely sliced
¼ cup roughly chopped flat-leaf parsley
½ cup fresh wholegrain breadcrumbs (made from
   day-old wholegrain bread)
canola oil spray
lime wedges

Sweet chilli mayonnaise
¼ cup sweet chilli sauce
½ cup fat-free mayonnaise
1 tablespoon lime juice

To make the sweet chilli mayonnaise, place all the mayonnaise ingredients in a bowl and mix well. Cover and set aside.

Boil the rice for 10–15 minutes until cooked, then drain. Place the rice, tuna, corn, coriander, egg whites, lime juice, spring onion and parsley in a large bowl and mix until well combined. Form the mixture into eight patties and flatten lightly with your hands. Place the breadcrumbs in a shallow dish. Sprinkle the patties with water and coat in the breadcrumbs, shaking off any excess.

Heat a large non-stick frying pan over medium heat and spray with canola oil. Cook the patties for 3 minutes each side or until cooked through. Serve with the mayonnaise, lime wedges and a green salad.

1 serve = 1 unit protein, 1 unit carbohydrates,
1 unit vegetables, 1 unit fats

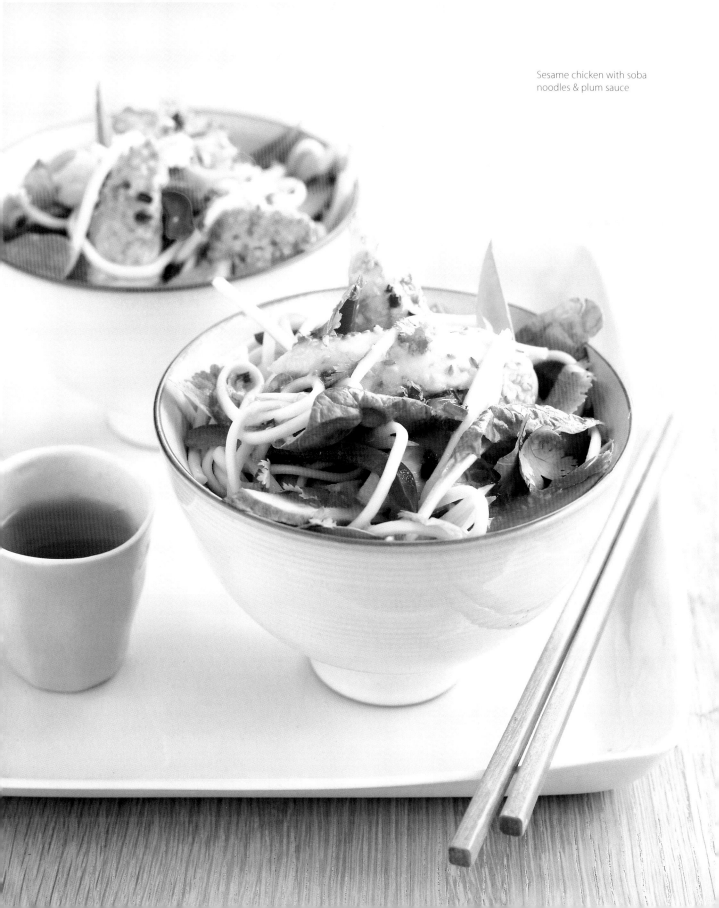

Sesame chicken with soba
noodles & plum sauce

Fennel & rosemary pork with wilted spinach & roast potatoes

Dinner Serves 4

- 600 g desiree potatoes (or sweet potatoes), peeled and quartered
- 2 tablespoons canola oil
- 2 cloves garlic, roughly chopped
- 2 teaspoons fennel seeds
- 2 teaspoons finely chopped rosemary
- 400 g pork fillet
- 1 tablespoon sterol spread
- 150 g baby spinach leaves
- 3 spring onions (scallions), finely sliced

Preheat the oven to 200°C and line a roasting tin with baking paper. Add the potatoes and 1 tablespoon of the canola oil, toss to coat and roast for 30 minutes.

Meanwhile, pound the garlic, fennel and rosemary in a mortar and pestle. Rub the mixture into the pork. Heat the remaining oil in a large heavy-based frying pan over medium heat, add the pork and cook for 3 minutes or until browned all over. Transfer to the roasting tin with the potatoes and roast for a further 15 minutes or until the potatoes are crisp and pork is cooked through. Remove the pork and potatoes to a plate, cover loosely with foil and allow to rest for 5 minutes. Reserve the pan juices.

Heat the sterol spread in a saucepan over medium heat and cook the spinach and spring onion for 2 minutes or until the spinach has wilted. Season with freshly ground black pepper and drizzle over the reserved pan juice. Cut the pork into thick slices and serve with the potatoes and spinach, plus steamed baby carrots.

1 serve = 1 unit protein, 1 unit carbohydrates, 1 unit vegetables, 3 units fats

Chicken dumpling & noodle soup with greens

Dinner Serves 4

- 2 litres salt-reduced chicken stock
- 1 × 3 cm piece ginger, finely shredded
- 320 g udon noodles
- 1 bunch choy sum, cut into 3 cm pieces
- 100 g snow peas, trimmed and finely sliced
- 1 packet baby corn, sliced
- 1 tablespoon salt-reduced soy sauce
- 3 spring onions (scallions), finely sliced on an angle
- 1 red chilli, seeded and finely sliced
- ¼ cup roughly chopped coriander

Chicken dumplings
- 400 g lean minced chicken
- 2 spring onions (scallions), finely sliced
- 1 clove garlic, crushed
- 5 water chestnuts, finely chopped
- 1 tablespoon salt-reduced soy sauce
- 1 tablespoon cornflour

To make the dumplings, place all the dumpling ingredients in a bowl and mix until well combined. Roll into 20 even balls.

Place the stock and ginger in a large saucepan and bring to the boil. Reduce heat and simmer for 5 minutes. Bring the stock back to the boil and add the dumplings. Simmer for 3 minutes or until they float, then remove and divide among four bowls.

Return the stock to the boil, add the noodles and cook for 5 minutes. Add the vegetables, soy sauce and spring onion and simmer for 30 seconds. Ladle the noodles, vegetables and stock over the dumplings and sprinkle with chilli and coriander. Serve immediately.

1 serve = 1 unit protein, 1 unit carbohydrates, 2 units vegetables

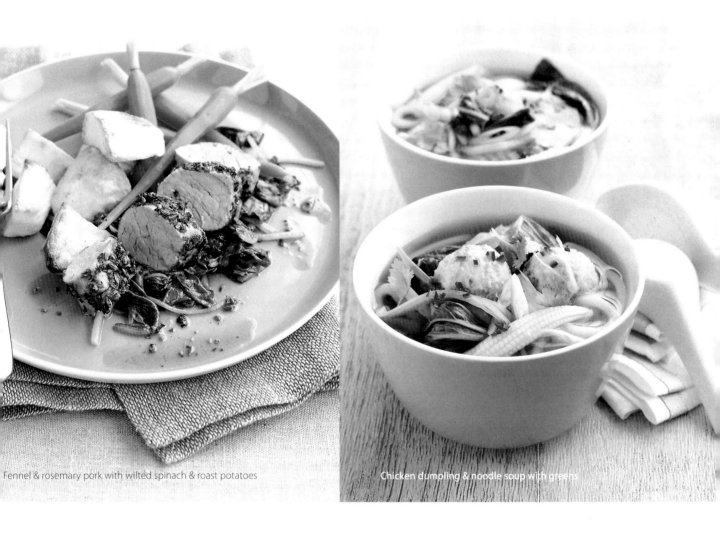

Fennel & rosemary pork with wilted spinach & roast potatoes

Chicken dumpling & noodle soup with greens

Indian pork curry with minted yoghurt & basmati rice

Dinner Serves 4

¾ cup basmati rice (makes approx 1⅓ cups cooked)
canola oil spray
400 g pork loin steaks, cut into 3 cm cubes
1 brown onion, finely chopped
1 clove garlic, crushed
3 tablespoons mild curry paste
1 × 400 g tin salt-reduced chopped tomatoes
½ cup salt-reduced beef stock
1 cup low-fat natural yoghurt
150 g green beans, trimmed and cut
    into 5 cm lengths
200 g cherry tomatoes, halved
⅓ cup roughly chopped coriander
⅓ cup shredded mint

Boiled the rice for 10–15 minutes until cooked. Drain and keep warm.

Meanwhile, heat a large saucepan over medium heat and spray with canola oil. Add half the pork and cook for 2–3 minutes or until browned. Remove from the pan and repeat with the remaining pork.

Add the onion and garlic to the pan and cook for 2 minutes or until softened. Stir in the curry paste and cook for a further minute until aromatic. Add the pork, chopped tomatoes and stock and simmer, covered, for 15 minutes or until the pork is tender.

Add the yoghurt, beans and cherry tomatoes and simmer, uncovered, for 2–3 minutes until the vegetables are tender. Stir in the coriander and mint and serve with basmati rice and green leafy vegetables.

1 serve = 1 unit protein, 1 unit carbohydrates,
2 units vegetables, 3 units fats

Slow-cooked lamb shanks with beans, carrots & spring onions

Dinner Serves 4

1 tablespoon canola oil
4 lamb shanks on the bone, French-trimmed
    (100 g meat per person)
2 cloves garlic, finely chopped
2 bunches spring onions (scallions), trimmed
    and sliced
2 carrots, peeled and sliced
2 sticks celery, sliced
3 cups salt-reduced beef stock
1 cup red wine
1 tablespoon salt-reduced tomato paste
1 teaspoon dried rosemary
¼ cup roughly chopped flat-leaf parsley
1 × 400 g tin salt-reduced cannellini beans,
    drained and rinsed

Preheat the oven to 200°C.

Heat the oil in a large heavy-based frying pan over high heat, add the shanks and cook for 5 minutes until well browned. Transfer to a deep ovenproof dish.

Add the garlic, spring onion, carrot and celery to the frying pan and cook for 3 minutes or until starting to colour. Stir in the stock, wine, tomato paste and rosemary and bring to the boil. Pour this mixture over the shanks, cover with foil and cook in the oven for 1½–2 hours or until the meat begins to fall off the bone.

Remove from the oven and stir in the parsley and cannellini beans. Return to the oven for 5 minutes to heat through, then serve with steamed vegetables.

1 serve = 1 unit protein, 1 unit carbohydrates,
1 unit vegetables, 1 unit fats

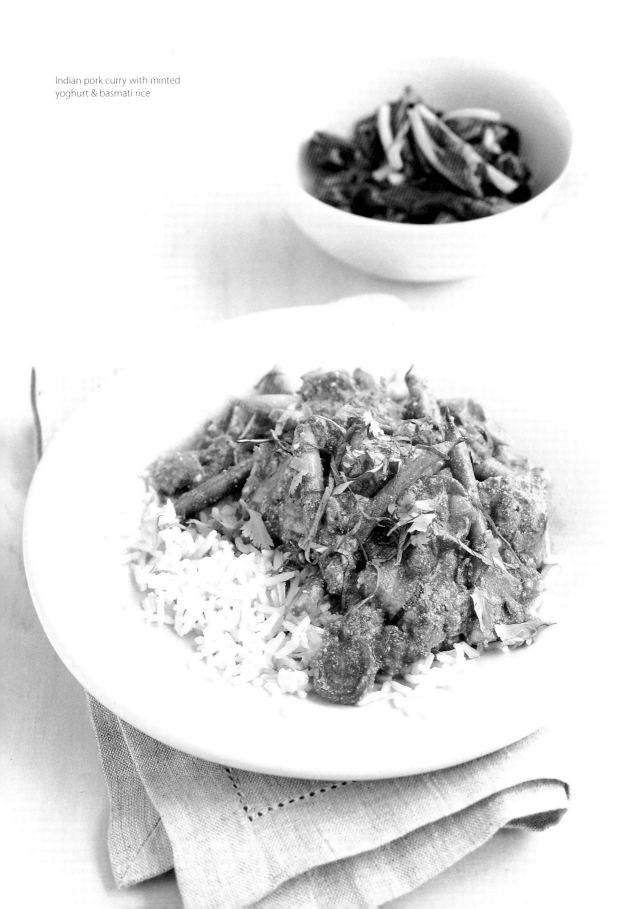

Indian pork curry with minted
yoghurt & basmati rice

Thyme & lemon lamb cutlets with zucchini & chickpea salad

Dinner Serves 4

80 g low-fat ricotta

1 tablespoon roughly chopped basil

2 teaspoons finely chopped lemon thyme

2 teaspoons olive oil

1 clove garlic, crushed

1 teaspoon finely grated lemon zest

1 tablespoon lemon juice

500 g lamb cutlets, trimmed of fat

olive oil spray

Zucchini & chickpea salad

2 zucchini, halved lengthways

olive oil spray

2 tablespoons pitted kalamata olives, halved

1 × 400 g tin salt-reduced chickpeas, drained and rinsed

1 cup roughly chopped flat-leaf parsley

1 bulb fennel, finely sliced

1 tablespoon olive oil

2 teaspoons balsamic vinegar

Combine the ricotta, basil, lemon thyme, olive oil, garlic, lemon zest and juice in a bowl and season with freshly ground black pepper.

Using a sharp knife, cut a slit into the side of each lamb cutlet (be careful not to cut all the way through). Place 2 teaspoons of the ricotta mixture into each cutlet, then press together with your fingers.

Heat a chargrill or barbecue to high. Lightly spray the cutlets with olive oil, then cook on the grill for 3–5 minutes each side or until cooked to your liking. Set aside on a plate, loosely covered in foil. Keep the chargrill or barbeque hot.

For the chickpea sald, lightly spray the zucchini with olive oil and cook on the chargrill or barbeque, cut-side down, for 5 minutes. Remove and cut into 3 cm pieces. Transfer to a bowl, toss with the remaining salad ingredients and serve with the lamb cutlets.

1 serve = 1 unit protein, 1 unit carbohydrates, ½ unit cheese, 1 unit vegetables, 1 unit fats

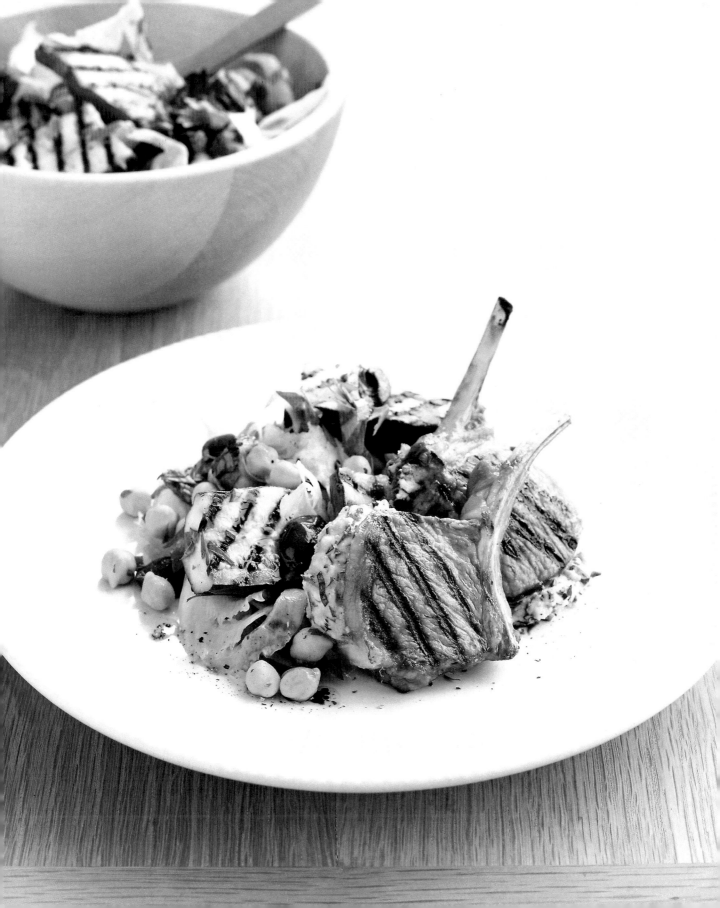

Beef & Guinness casserole

Dinner Serves 4

400 g beef, cut into 4 cm cubes

1 tablespoon wholemeal plain flour

2 tablespoons canola oil

2 brown onions, diced

2 carrots, peeled and thickly sliced

3 sticks celery, thickly sliced

2 tablespoons salt-reduced tomato paste

1 × 440 ml can Guinness

2 cups salt-reduced beef stock

1 bay leaf

5 cm sprig rosemary

5 cm sprig thyme

200 g small button mushrooms

600 g chat potatoes, halved

¼ cup roughly chopped flat-leaf parsley

Place the beef and flour in a bowl and season with pepper. Toss the beef through the flour, shaking off any excess. Heat 1 tablespoon of the oil in a heavy flameproof casserole dish over medium heat. Add the beef in batches and cook for 3 minutes or until browned. Remove and set aside.

Add the remaining oil to the casserole dish and cook the onion, carrot and celery for 5 minutes until they begin to soften. Stir in the tomato paste and cook for 1 minute. Add the beef, Guinness, stock, bay leaf, rosemary and thyme. Bring to the boil, then reduce the heat and simmer, covered, for 1½ hours, stirring occasionally. Add the mushrooms and potatoes and simmer, uncovered, for a further 10–15 minutes. Stir in the parsley and serve with steamed green beans and broccolini.

1 serve = 1 unit protein, 1 unit carbohydrates,
1 unit vegetables, 2 units fats, ½ unit indulgence

Chargrilled steak sandwiches with tomato relish

Dinner Serves 4

1 tablespoon sterol spread

4 red onions, finely sliced

2 teaspoons salt-reduced Worcestershire sauce

4 × 100 g minute steaks

4 slices wholegrain bread, lightly toasted

8 baby cos lettuce leaves

1 × 225 g tin salt-reduced sliced beetroot, drained

4 tablespoons salt-reduced tomato relish

Heat the sterol spread in a saucepan over medium heat and cook the onion for 2 minutes or until starting to soften. Add the Worcestershire sauce and ¼ cup water and simmer for 10 minutes or until the liquid has been absorbed and the onion is golden and caramelised.

Heat a chargrill or barbecue to high. Cook the steaks for 1 minute each side, then remove to a plate and allow to rest for 1 minute.

Put a piece of toast on each serving plate and top with lettuce leaves and beetroot, then the steak, caramelised onion and a dollop of tomato relish. Serve immediately.

1 serve = 1 unit protein, 1 unit carbohydrates,
1 unit vegetables, 1 unit fats

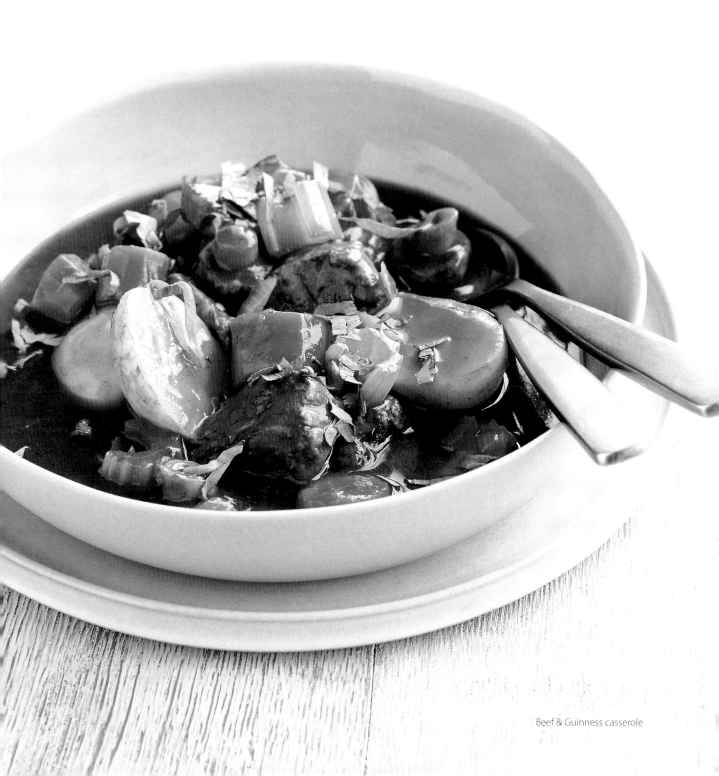

Beef & Guinness casserole

Dinner for 4

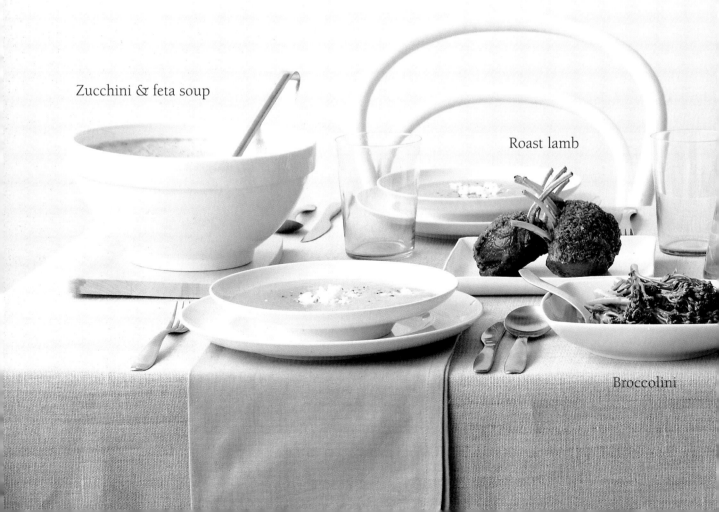

Zucchini & feta soup

Roast lamb

Broccolini

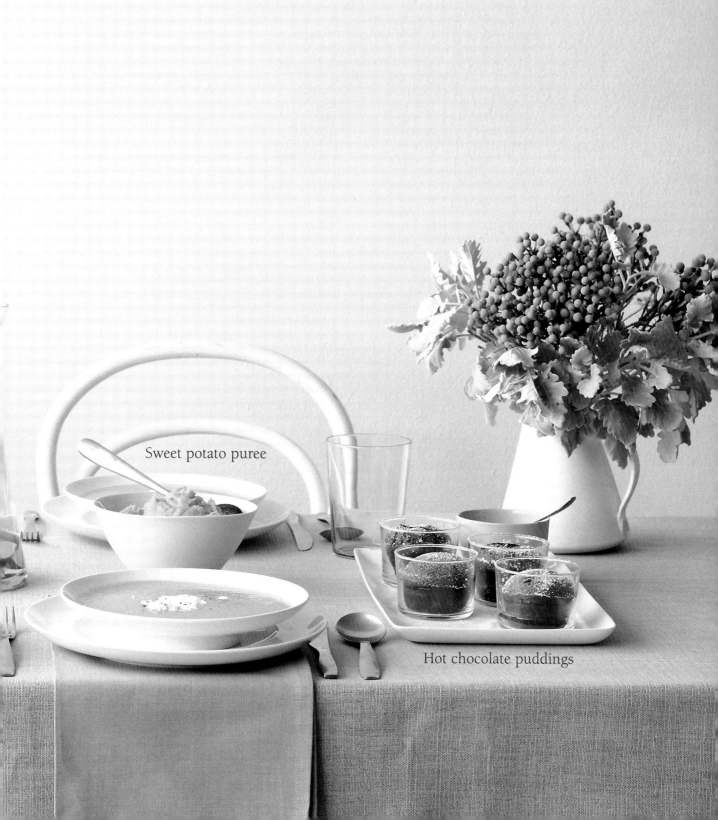

Sweet potato puree

Hot chocolate puddings

Zucchini & feta soup

2 tablespoons olive oil

1 brown onion, finely diced

1 clove garlic, crushed

1 tablespoon roughly chopped thyme

1 litre salt-reduced chicken stock

3 desiree potatoes, peeled and cut into
    1.5 cm cubes

4 large zucchini, cut into 1 cm slices

½ cup roughly chopped flat-leaf parsley

½ cup roughly chopped basil

¼ cup low-fat natural yoghurt

100 g low-fat, salt-reduced feta, crumbled

Heat the oil in a large saucepan over medium heat and cook the onion, garlic and thyme for 1 minute or until softened. Add the stock and potatoes, bring to the boil, then reduce the heat and simmer for 10 minutes or until the potato is tender. Add the zucchini and cook for a further 2 minutes or until soft. Stir in the parsley, basil and yoghurt.

Working in batches, transfer the soup to a food processor and season well with freshly ground black pepper. Puree the soup, ladle into bowls and sprinkle with the crumbled feta.

1 serve = ½ unit carbohydrates, ½ unit cheese

Roast lamb with sweet potato

2 tablespoons fresh wholemeal breadcrumbs
    (made from day-old wholemeal bread)

¼ cup roughly chopped flat-leaf parsley

1 tablespoon roughly chopped oregano

2 teaspoons roughly chopped rosemary

1 clove garlic, roughly chopped

1 tablespoon finely grated lemon zest

2 teaspoons olive oil

400 g racks of lamb, trimmed

canola oil spray

1 bunch broccolini, trimmed

Sweet potato puree

400 g sweet potatoes, peeled and
    cut into 2–3 cm cubes

1 tablespoon honey

1 tablespoon sterol spread

¼ cup low-fat sterol milk

Preheat the oven to 200°C. Place the breadcrumbs, herbs, garlic, zest, olive oil and some pepper in a food processor and whiz until the herbs are finely chopped. Firmly press the mixture onto one side of each rack of lamb.

Heat a large non-stick frying pan over medium heat and lightly spray with canola oil. Cook the lamb, crust-side up, for 2 minutes, then place in a baking dish and roast for 8–10 minutes for medium or until cooked to your liking. Remove from the oven, cover loosely with foil and allow to rest for 6 minutes.

To make the puree, place the sweet potato in a large saucepan of cold water and bring to the boil. Reduce the heat and simmer for 10 minutes, until the sweet potato is soft. Drain, then place in a food processor with the remaining ingredients and whiz until smooth. Season with pepper.

Meanwhile, bring a saucepan of water to the boil, add the broccolini and cook for 2 minutes. Drain well. Slice the lamb and serve with the broccolini and sweet potato puree.

1 serve = 1 unit protein, ½ unit carbohydrates, 1 unit fats

Hot chocolate puddings

canola oil spray

100 g dark chocolate (70% cocoa),
    broken into pieces

100 g sterol spread

4 eggs

¼ cup brown sugar

3 tablespoons wholemeal plain flour

icing sugar

low-fat sterol vanilla yoghurt

Preheat the oven to 180°C and lightly spray four 250 ml dariole moulds with canola oil.

Place the chocolate and sterol spread in a clean glass bowl and microwave on high for 30–40 seconds or until melted. Stir with a metal spoon until smooth.

Using electric beaters, beat the eggs and sugar on high for 5 minutes or until thick and the volume has doubled. Fold in the flour, then spoon the mixture into the dariole moulds. Place on a baking tray and bake for 8–10 minutes until just set (they should be puffed but still soft in the centre). Set aside for 2 minutes.

Lightly dust the puddings with icing sugar and serve with vanilla yoghurt.

1 serve = ½ unit protein, 1 unit dairy, 5 units fats,
2 units indulgence

Unit totals for dinner party: 1 unit carbohydrates,
1½ units protein, 1 unit dairy, ½ unit cheese, 6 units fats,
2 units indulgence

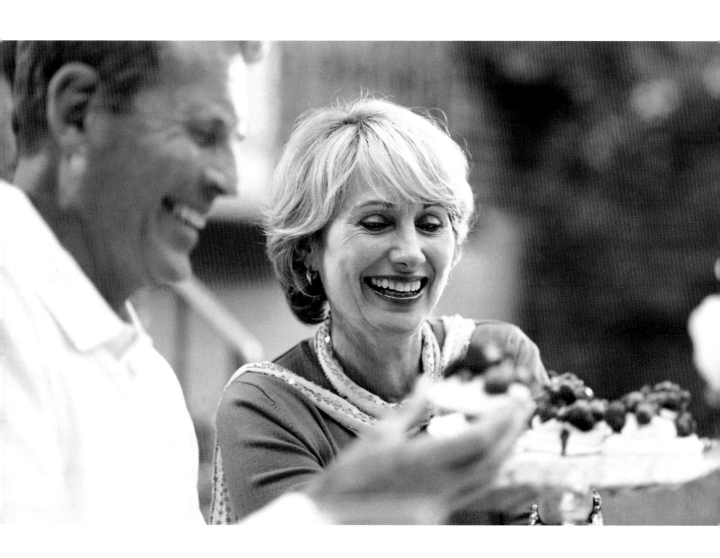

Desserts

Poached stone fruit with yoghurt

Dessert Serves 4

1 cup apple juice

1 cup water

1 stick cinnamon

1 vanilla bean, halved lengthways,
or ½ teaspoon vanilla bean paste

4 ripe nectarines or peaches

4 tablespoons low-fat natural yoghurt

4 tablespoons flaked almonds, lightly toasted

Combine the apple juice, water, cinnamon and vanilla in a saucepan and bring to the boil. Reduce the heat and simmer for 5 minutes. Add the fruit, bring to a simmer, then remove the pan from the heat and set aside for 10 minutes. Remove the cinnamon stick and the vanilla bean.

Divide the fruit and syrup among serving bowls, top with a dollop of yoghurt and sprinkle with flaked almonds.

1 serve = 1 unit fruit, ½ unit nuts *or* 2 units indulgence

Raspberry jelly with custard

Dessert Serves 6

85 g packet low-joule raspberry jelly crystals

1 cup clear apple juice

300 g frozen raspberries (no need to thaw)

low-fat custard

Place the jelly crystals in a heatproof jug, add 1 cup boiling water and stir until thoroughly dissolved. Add the apple juice and stir well.

Put 50 g of the frozen berries in each of 6 × 125 ml plastic dariole moulds or jelly moulds. Pour the jelly mixture over the top. Place the moulds on a tray and refrigerate for 4 hours or until set.

Run the bottom of the moulds under warm water to loosen, then turn out onto serving plates. Serve with custard.

1 serve = 1 unit dairy, ½ unit fruit

Note: You can buy low-fat custard ready-made or make your own with custard powder and sterol milk.

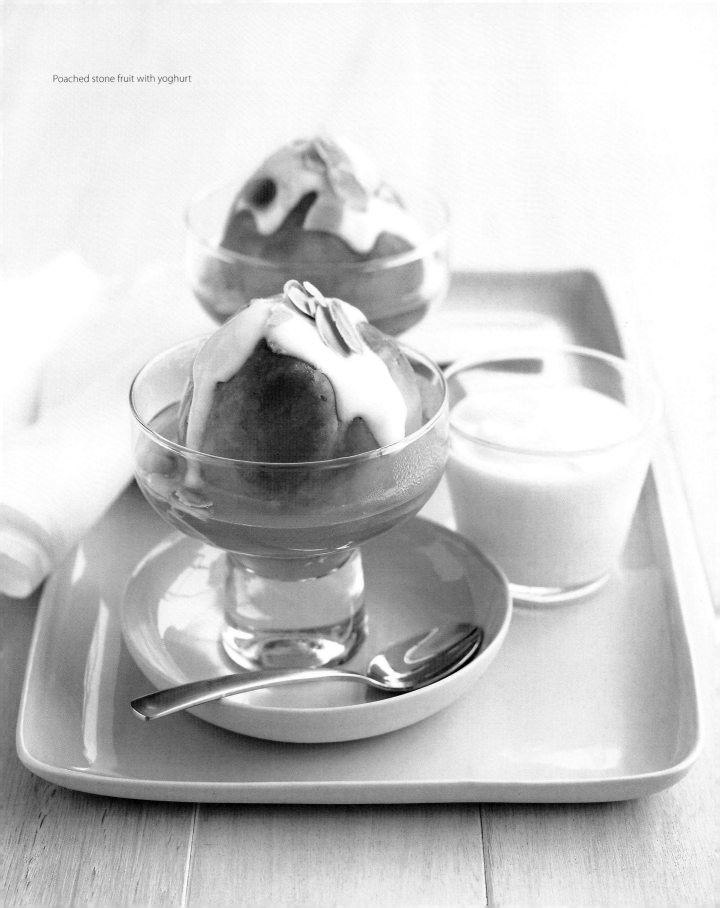

Poached stone fruit with yoghurt

Plum & hazelnut crumble

Dessert Serves 8–10

> 1 × 200 g tin apple pie fruit
> 825 g tinned plums in natural juice, drained,
>   reserving 1 cup juice, and stones removed
> ½ cup wholemeal plain flour
> 2 tablespoons brown sugar
> ¾ cup rolled oats
> ½ cup ground hazelnuts
> 3 tablespoons sterol spread
> low-fat custard (optional)

Preheat the oven to 200°C. Place the apple, plums and reserved juice in a large bowl and gently fold them together. Spoon into a 1.5 litre ceramic ovenproof dish.

Place the flour, sugar, oats and hazelnuts in a bowl and rub in the sterol spread until the mixture resembles breadcrumbs. Spoon the crumble topping over the fruit and bake for 20 minutes or until golden. Serve with custard, if desired.

1 serve = 2 units indulgence + 1 unit dairy if you have custard

Note: You can buy low-fat custard ready-made or make your own with custard powder and sterol milk.

Chocolate pots

Dessert Serves 4

> 100 g dark chocolate (70% cocoa), broken into pieces
> 200 ml sterol vanilla yoghurt
> 1 teaspoon vanilla extract
> raspberries
> icing sugar

Place the chocolate in a heatproof bowl. Set over a saucepan of gently simmering water, ensuring the bottom of the bowl does not touch the water. Add 1 tablespoon hot water and stir with a metal spoon until the chocolate is melted and the mixture is smooth.

Add the yoghurt and vanilla to the chocolate mixture, then spoon into four 125 ml serving bowls. Place the bowls on a tray and refrigerate for 10 minutes.

To serve, top with fresh raspberries and dust with icing sugar.

1 serve = 1½ units indulgence

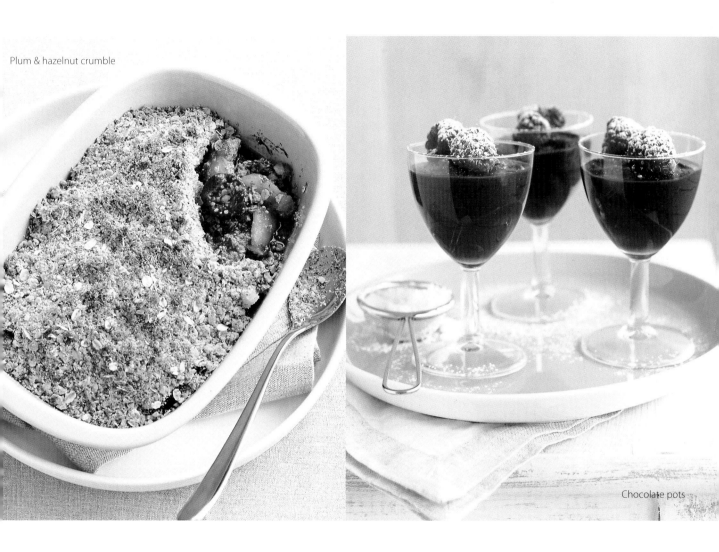

Plum & hazelnut crumble

Chocolate pots

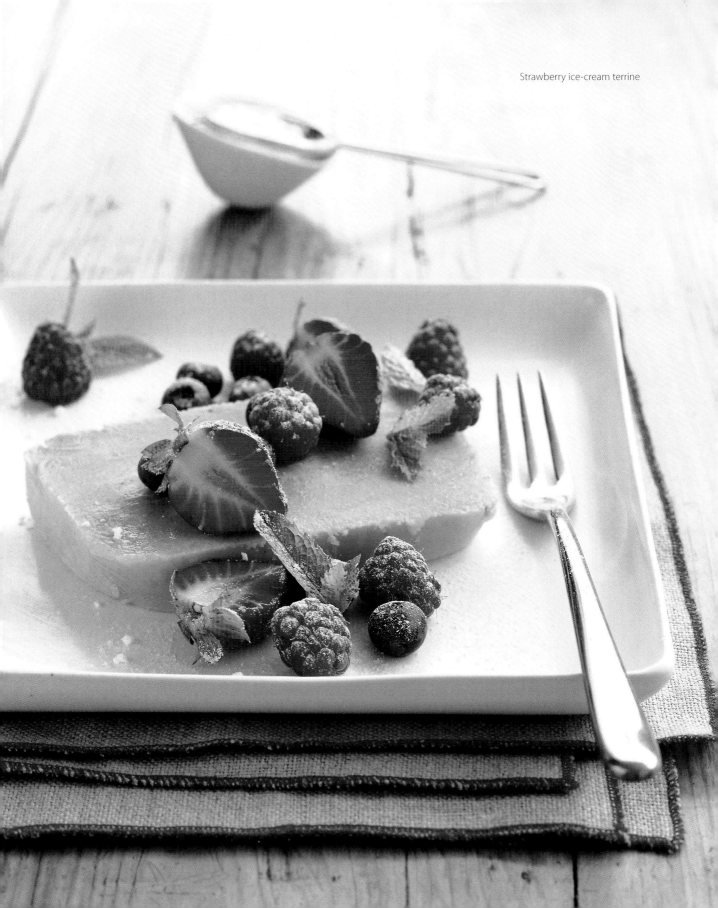

Strawberry ice-cream terrine

Strawberry ice-cream terrine

Dessert Serves 6

500 g strawberries, hulled and coarsely chopped

1 tablespoon Equal or other powdered sweetener

1 kg sterol vanilla yoghurt

2 tablespoons custard powder

2 cups low-fat sterol milk

icing sugar

mixed berries

mint leaves

Line a loaf tin with plastic wrap, leaving a 5 cm overhang.

Combine the strawberries and sweetener in a saucepan over low heat and cook for 3 minutes or until the sweetener has dissolved and the strawberries have started to soften. Strain the mixture through a sieve into a large bowl, pushing the berries with the back of a spoon. Discard the seeds. Fold the yoghurt into the syrup.

Place the custard powder in a small bowl and mix with enough milk to make a smooth paste. Stir the paste into the remaining milk and pour into a clean saucepan. Stir constantly over low heat for about 3 minutes until the custard has thickened. Set aside to cool slightly.

Stir the custard into the strawberry mixture and pour into the loaf tin. Cover with plastic wrap and place in the freezer for 4 hours or overnight to set. Cut into slices, dust with icing sugar, and serve with mixed berries and mint leaves.

1 serve = ½ unit fruit, 1 unit dairy

Apple & almond strudel

Dessert Serves 6

1 × 400 g tin apple pie fruit

3 tablespoons sultanas

½ teaspoon ground cinnamon

½ teaspoon ground cloves

1 tablespoon Equal or other powdered sweetener

5 sheets filo pastry

canola oil spray

¼ cup almond meal

icing sugar

low-fat custard or yoghurt

Preheat the oven to 200°C and line a baking tray with baking paper.

Place the apple, sultanas, cinnamon, cloves and sweetener in a bowl and mix well.

Lay out a sheet of filo on a clean work surface, lightly spray with canola oil and sprinkle with almond meal. Repeat with the remaining filo, spraying with oil and adding almond meal to make five layers.

Spoon the apple mixture along the long edge of the pastry, leaving a 5 cm border. Fold in the ends and roll to enclose the filling. Place on the baking tray, seam-side down, and spray with canola oil. Bake for 30 minutes or until golden.

Dust with icing sugar and serve warm with low-fat custard or yoghurt.

1 serve = 1 unit indulgence

Wholemeal lemon crepes with raspberries

Dessert Serves 4

    1 cup wholemeal self-raising flour
    1 egg
    2 egg whites
    1½ cups low-fat sterol milk
    1 tablespoon finely grated lemon zest
    canola oil spray
    200 g vanilla sterol yoghurt mixed
        with a drizzle of honey
    1 punnet raspberries
    icing sugar

Whisk together the flour, egg, egg whites, milk and zest. Set aside for 10 minutes to rest.

Heat a small non-stick frying pan over medium heat and lightly spray with canola oil. Spoon ¼ cup of mixture into the pan and swirl to cover the base, pouring off any excess. Cook for 1 minute or until the edges are crisp. Flip over and cook the other side for 20 seconds. Remove from the pan and keep warm. Repeat with the remaining mixture to make eight crepes.

Arrange the crepes on serving plates and top with a dollop of yoghurt and some fresh raspberries. Dust with icing sugar just before serving.

1 serve = ½ unit fruit, 2 units indulgence

Papaya & strawberry fruit plate with passionfruit & orange

Dessert Serves 6

    1 papaya, peeled, seeded and sliced
    2 oranges, peeled and cut into rounds
    1 punnet strawberries, hulled and halved
    3 passionfruit, halved
    ¼ cup mint leaves
    low-fat sterol vanilla yoghurt

Arrange the papaya, oranges and strawberries on a serving platter. Dot the passionfruit halves around the platter and sprinkle with mint leaves.

Serve with vanilla yoghurt.

1 serve = 1 unit dairy, 2 units fruit

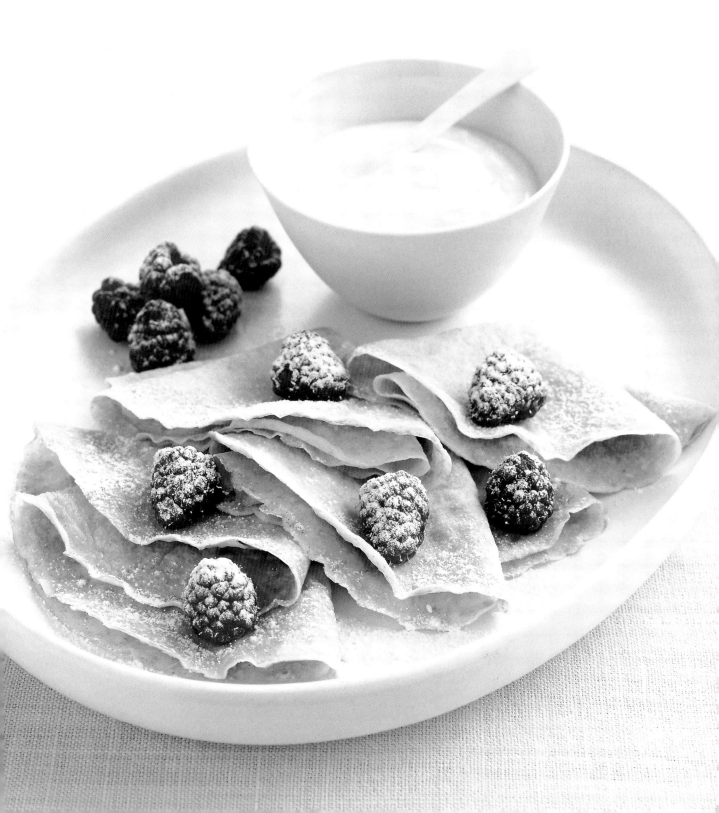

Wholemeal lemon crepes with raspberries

Cocktail party for 8

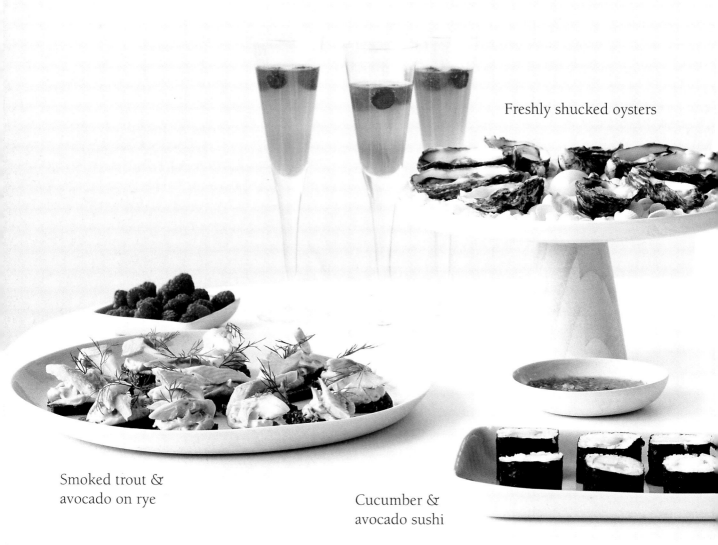

Champagne cocktail

Freshly shucked oysters

Smoked trout &
avocado on rye

Cucumber &
avocado sushi

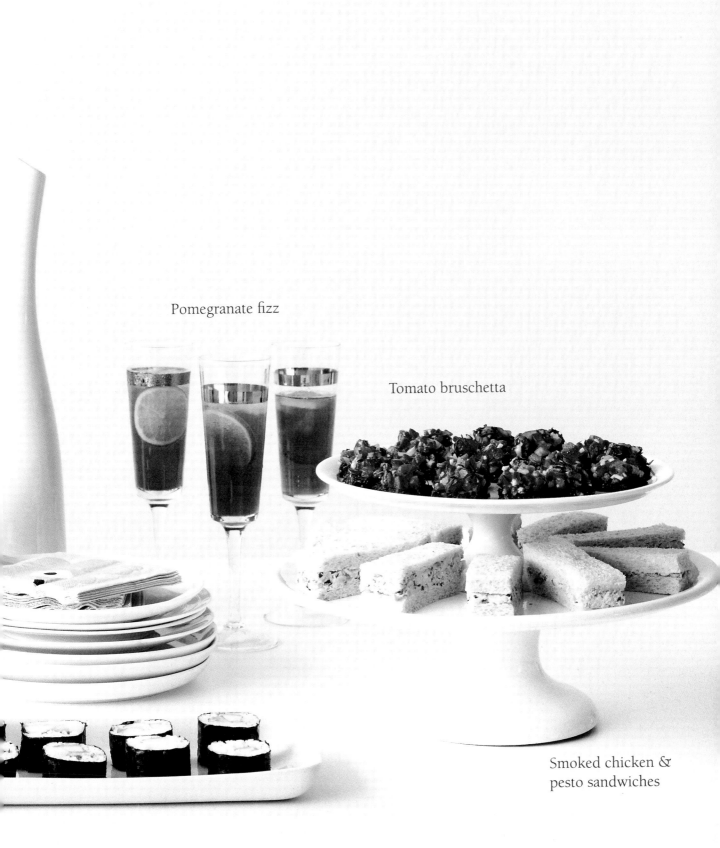

Pomegranate fizz

Tomato bruschetta

Smoked chicken &
pesto sandwiches

Smoked trout & avocado on rye

Makes 16

    1 avocado, peeled, stone removed
    2 tablespoons lemon juice
    splash of Tabasco sauce
    1 tablespoon grated fresh horseradish
    1 tablespoon finely chopped chives
    4 slices rye bread, toasted, cut into quarters
    160 g piece hot-smoked trout (see note on
        page 158), flaked
    16 sprigs dill

Place the avocado, lemon juice, Tabasco sauce and horseradish in a food processor and whiz until smooth. Stir in the chives.

Spoon the avocado mixture onto the rye toasts, top with a chunk of trout and garnish with a dill sprig.

Smoked chicken & pesto sandwiches

Makes 12

    300 g smoked or barbecued skinless chicken breast
    ½ cup low-fat ricotta
    1 tablespoon pesto
    1 tablespoon pine nuts, lightly toasted and
        roughly chopped
    ½ cup baby rocket, roughly chopped
    8 slices wholemeal sandwich bread

Finely chop the chicken breast and place in a bowl with the ricotta, pesto, pine nuts and rocket. Mix well and spread over four slices of bread. Top with the remaining bread slices.

Using a sharp serrated knife, trim the crusts off each sandwich, then cut each into three fingers.

Cucumber & avocado sushi

Makes 16

    ½ cup medium-grain rice
    2 tablespoons rice-wine vinegar or sushi seasoning
    4 sheets nori
    1 avocado, peeled and sliced
    1 Lebanese cucumber, cut into 1 cm thick batons
    wasabi
    soy sauce
    pickled ginger

Place the rice and 1 cup water in a small saucepan and bring to the boil. Reduce the heat and simmer, covered, for 10 minutes. Remove from heat and stand, covered, for 10 minutes. Pour the vinegar over the rice and gently turn with a spoon. Cover with paper towel until cool.

Place a sheet of nori on a clean dry surface. Place 2 tablespoons rice along the edge of the sheet then, with damp fingers, push the rice out to a thickness of 1 cm. Place strips of avocado and cucumber along the rice and roll tightly. Seal the edges with a little water. Cut each roll into four with a sharp serrated knife and serve with wasabi, soy sauce and pickled ginger.

Freshly shucked oysters

Makes 24

    1 tablespoon finely diced golden shallots
    1 tablespoon red-wine vinegar
    2 dozen rock oysters, freshly shucked
    crushed ice
    lemon wedges

Mix the shallots and vinegar together in a small bowl and season with freshly ground black pepper.

Arrange the oysters on crushed ice on a platter, drizzle with the dressing and serve with lemon wedges. Make sure the oysters are super-cold.

Tomato bruschetta

Makes 20

- 5 slices rye bread, crusts removed and cut into quarters
- olive oil spray
- 2 vine-ripened tomatoes, finely diced
- 1 roasted capsicum, finely diced
- 2 cloves garlic, finely chopped
- 1 small red onion, finely diced
- 1 tablespoon roughly chopped flat-leaf parsley
- 1 tablespoon shredded basil
- 1 tablespoon olive oil

Preheat the oven to 200°C. Lightly spray the bread with olive oil, place on a baking tray and bake for 10 minutes or until golden and crisp. Remove from oven and set aside to cool completely.

Mix together the remaining ingredients and season with freshly ground black pepper. Spoon the tomato mixture onto the rye toasts and serve immediately.

Champagne cocktail

Makes 8

- 240 ml guava juice
- 16 raspberries
- champagne

Pour 30 ml guava juice into the bottom of each glass. Drop in two raspberries, then fill to the top with champagne.

Pomegranate fizz

- pomegranate juice
- soda water
- thin slices of lime

Pour equal portions of pomegranate juice and soda water into each champagne flute. Garnish with a thin slice of lime.

Unit totals for cocktail party: 1 unit protein,
1 unit carbohydrates, 1 unit fruit, 2 units fats, 1 unit indulgence

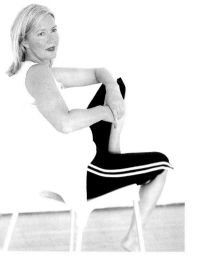

Glossary

Antioxidant

A substance found in food that inactivates certain cell-damaging compounds called free radicals. Free radicals have been linked to conditions such as CVD and cancer. Common antioxidants include vitamin E, vitamin C and beta-carotene.

Carbohydrate

One of the three main nutrients in food (the others are *protein* and *fat*). Foods that provide carbohydrate are breads, cereals, legumes, whole grains, vegetables, fruit, some dairy products and sugars.

Cardiac risk factors

Factors that can increase your risk of developing CVD. Some can't be changed, such as age, gender or family history. Those that can be changed include poor nutrition, smoking, high blood cholesterol, lack of exercise, excess weight, obesity, high blood pressure and diabetes.

Cardiovascular disease (CVD)

A class of conditions involving the blood vessels (arteries and veins) of the heart, brain and body. Examples include heart attack and stroke.

Cholesterol

A compound needed in small amounts by the body for good cell health and hormone production. Too much cholesterol in the blood can increase your risk of CVD. It is made by the liver and obtained from animal products such as offal, fatty meats, full-fat dairy products and egg yolks. Eating saturated or trans fats reduces the clearance of cholesterol from the blood by the liver and causes a rise of cholesterol levels in the bloodstream.

Cholesterol – high-density lipoprotein (HDL)

A healthy compound in the body that transports cholesterol away from the arteries and, if elevated, can reduce the risk of cardiovascular disease.

Cholesterol – low-density lipoprotein (LDL)

An unhealthy compound in the body that transports cholesterol in the blood, which, if elevated, can increase risk of CVD.

Cholesterol – total cholesterol (TC)

The total amount of cholesterol in the blood, which, if elevated, can increase the risk of CVD.

CLIP

The Complete Lifestyle Program. A total diet and exercise program for lowering cholesterol and reducing the risk of CVD.

Energy

Another word for kilojoules or calories. Energy comes from four sources in food and drink: fat, carbohydrate, protein and alcohol. For your weight to remain stable, the amount of energy you get from food and drink needs to be equal to the amount of energy you use in physical activity and maintenance of bodily functions.

Fat

One of the three main nutrients, fat is present in oils, butter, margarine, eggs, nuts, avocado, full-fat dairy foods, biscuits, cakes, pastry and fatty meats. There are 3 main types of fat: *monounsaturated, polyunsaturated* and *saturated.*

Fat – monounsaturated

Mainly found in margarine spreads and oils (such as olive, canola and peanut oils), avocados and some nuts. This type of fat is neutral or slightly lowers blood LDL cholesterol levels.

Fat – polyunsaturated

Found mainly in margarine spreads and oils (such as sunflower, soybean and safflower oils), fish, and some nuts and seeds. This type of fat lowers blood LDL cholesterol levels. See also *Omega-3 fatty acid.*

Fat – saturated

Found mainly in butter, meat, animal skin and full-fat dairy foods. It also occurs in two vegetable oils, palm oil and coconut oil. It raises blood LDL cholesterol levels.

Fat – trans

A type of poly- or monounsaturated fat that, because of its chemical structure, behaves more like a saturated fat in the body.

Fatty acid

One of the building blocks of fats and oils, and the basis of fatty acids chains of carbon atoms. The length of the chains and how the carbon atoms are linked to each other can determine the health properties of the fatty acid. See also *Omega-3 fatty acid.*

Fibre

A substance not digested by the body and found in plant foods such as breads, cereals, whole grains, fruits, vegetables, legumes and nuts. Fibre can be split into two main groups – *soluble fibre* and *insoluble fibre.* The main role of fibre is to promote healthy bowel function by giving bulk to your stool and preventing constipation. Consumption of fibre from whole grains is associated with lower CVD risk. Consumption of soluble fibre is associated with a lower LDL cholesterol level.

Glycaemic Index (GI)

A ranking system for *carbohydrate* food sources based on their effect on blood sugar levels. The lower the GI, the longer the body takes to break down and release the *carbohydrate* from the food into the body.

Insoluble fibre

A type of dietary fibre that does not dissolve in water. It can be found in wholegrain foods, the skins of fruit and vegetables, nuts, seeds and beans. See also *Fibre.*

Insulin resistance (IR)
A condition in which the body's cells are less responsive to the actions of normal amounts of insulin. It can occur in people who are older, overweight or have type 2 diabetes.

Legume
The general name given to dried and tinned beans, peas and lentils. Common varieties include chickpeas, kidney beans, baked beans and bean mixes, split peas, soybeans and lentils (red, green or brown). Legumes are also called pulses.

Metabolic syndrome
A condition linked to an increased risk of CVD and type 2 diabetes, with the presence of at least three of the following factors: excess abdominal fat, high *triglyceride* levels, high blood pressure, low HDL-cholesterol levels, insulin resistance.

Omega-3 fatty acid
A type of polyunsaturated fat that can be long-chain (LC), such as those in fish oil, or short-chain (SC), from plants such as canola and linseed. LC omega-3 fatty acids have been shown to reduce the risk of sudden death from heart attack.

Plant sterols
Plant compounds that have a similar structure to dietary cholesterols and that compete with them for absorption in the body. Consuming enough plant sterols can lower your blood cholesterol levels.

Polyphenols
A group of plant-based compounds with antioxidant properties. Common examples include tannins in tea and flavonoids in cocoa and cocoa products.

Protein
One of the three main nutrients in food, along with *carbohydrate* and *fat*. Foods that provide protein include lean red and white meat, fish, eggs, low-fat dairy foods, legumes and nuts.

Soluble fibre
The type of dietary fibre that dissolves in water and is more digestible. It has a gel-like consistency and is found in fruit, legumes (e.g. chickpeas and lentils) and cereals (e.g. oats and barley). See also *Fibre*.

Triglyceride
A type of fat found in the blood, which, if elevated, can increase risk of CVD.

Vascular
A term that refers to blood vessels (particularly arteries).

Appendix 1

Assessing your aerobic fitness

Warning

The following information is for general guidance only and should not be treated as a substitute for medical advice from a health-care professional. It is important that you consult your doctor and obtain medical clearance before undertaking any form of strenuous physical activity or attempting to do this fitness test. Remember, if it hurts or you feel dizzy, nauseous or light-headed, experience chest pain or simply feel you can't go any further, stop immediately.

3-minute step test

You can determine your level of aerobic fitness (which is important for overall health) by assessing your heart's ability to recover from exercise, using a simple 3-minute step test. This can act as a benchmark for future testing. After performing the test, undertake the exercise program for a few months and then do the test again to compare the results and monitor your progress.

It is not always possible to do the test exactly as described. The important point is that you are consistent and do the test exactly the same way each time so you can compare your scores. The table of results is only a guide and is based on the test being performed a specific way, and may not be exactly accurate if modified in any way. Don't worry about this; the important thing is that you improve your own score.

Equipment required

1　A 30-centimetre-high step (for example a solid chair, bench or box). Check that it is stable before you start the test. Alternatively, use the bottom step of a staircase in your house. If your stairs don't measure 30 centimetres, you could put together some sturdy boards to the approximate height.
2　A watch with a second hand, or a stopwatch.
3　Comfortable exercise clothes and appropriate walking shoes.

Performing the test

The step test can be quite demanding, so if you are out of shape or think the test might be too hard for you, take a 1-minute pre-test to see how you feel. If you cannot finish the 3-minute test, it means that your fitness levels are very low and you should consult your doctor before undertaking any further strenuous exercise. You should not perform this test if you are taking beta-blockers or any other medication that affects your heart rate.

1　Stand in front of the bench.
2　Step on and off the bench for 3 minutes. Step up with one foot (your leading foot) and then the other foot until you are standing on the bench, then step down again, leading with the same foot. Don't rush; try to maintain a steady, four-beat cycle. This is easier if you say to yourself 'up, up, down, down'. You should aim for 24 completed

steps up and down per minute (96 single steps) to ensure you are stepping at the correct pace. To do this, use the second hand of your watch to ensure that you complete approximately 6 of the up-up-down-down sequences in 15 seconds. (You may want to practise this before taking the actual test.) It might help to have someone count for you and monitor the time so that you can concentrate on stepping.

3   Continue the test for 3 minutes.

4   At the end of 3 minutes, immediately sit down, find your pulse and record your heart rate (see method below) for 1 minute. You should start recording within 5 seconds of stopping. Ensure you start counting at zero. In contrast to taking your pulse during exercise, you must count your pulse for the whole minute.

5   Your score is the total number of heart beats counted in the 1-minute recovery period.

6   Compare your score with the figures in the chart opposite to determine your fitness category. Note that there are separate charts for men and women. As you become fitter, your score will decrease.

The test results can be altered by environmental (heat and humidity), dietary (time since your last meal) and behavioural (smoking or previous activity) factors. To control for these factors, take the test in the same way and at the same time of day each time.

Determining your pulse rate (manual method)

Practise finding and counting your pulse *before* you start the test. The most convenient place to measure your pulse is at your radial artery. To measure your pulse, press your index and middle fingers (*do not* use your thumb) firmly onto the wrist of your opposite hand, about 2 centimetres down from the base of your thumb. When you find a pulse, count the number of beats within a 1-minute period.

If you are having trouble finding the pulse in your wrist, you could measure the pulse in your carotid artery at the side of the neck, just under your jawbone. Make sure you don't press too hard or your measurement will be inaccurate.

Recovery heart-rate scores for men after the 3-minute step test

fitness level	age group					
	18–25	26–35	36–45	46–55	56–65	65+
excellent	less than 79	less than 81	less than 83	less than 87	less than 86	less than 88
good	79–89	81–89	83–96	87–97	86–97	88–96
above average	90–99	90–99	97–103	98–105	98–103	97–103
average	100–105	100–107	104–112	106–116	104–112	104–113
below average	106–116	108–117	113–119	117–122	113–120	114–120
poor	117–128	118–128	120–130	123–132	121–129	121–130
very poor	more than 128	more than 128	more than 130	more than 132	more than 129	more than 130

Recovery heart-rate scores for women after the 3-minute step test

fitness level	age group					
	18–25	26–35	36–45	46–55	56–65	65+
excellent	less than 85	less than 88	less than 90	less than 94	less than 95	less than 90
good	85–98	88–99	90–102	95–104	95–104	90–102
above average	99–108	100–111	103–110	105–115	105–112	103–115
average	109–117	112–119	111–118	116–120	113–118	116–122
below average	118–126	120–128	119–128	121–126	119–128	123–128
poor	127–140	129–138	129–140	127–135	129–139	129–134
very poor	more than 140	more than 138	more than 140	more than 135	more than 139	more than 134

Adapted from L. Golding, C. Myers & W. Sinning, *Y's Way to Physical Fitness*, Human Kinetics Publishing, Champaign, Illinois, 1989.

Appendix 2

Daily activity checklist

Monday (example)	Tuesday	Wednesday	Thursday	Friday	Saturday	Sunday
park the car further away from work and walk briskly (10 minutes)						
replace a coffee break with a 'walk and talk' around the block with colleagues (10 minutes)						
briskly walk back to the car after work (10 minutes)						
play footy with the kids after work (20 minutes)						
total time: 50 minutes						

Walking program

Here is the walking program we recommend if you are just starting to get active.

Suggested walking program

training week	frequency (days a week)	intensity (target zone)	duration (minutes per session)
1	3	1	20–30
2	3	1	20–30
3	3	2	20–30
4	3	2	30–40
5	3	2	30–40
6	4	2	30–40
7	4	2	45–60
8	5	2	45–60
9	5	2	45–60
10	5	3	45–60
11	5	3	45–60
12	5	3	45–60

Make copies of the checklist below (or download it from our website www.csiro.au/clip) and fill it out for the days you walk each week.

WEEK:

	Monday	Tuesday	Wednesday	Thursday	Friday	Saturday	Sunday
warm up (Y/N)							
duration of session (minutes)							
intensity of session (target zone)							
heart rate							
cool down (Y/N)							
thoughts & feelings							
wellbeing							

Muscle-strengthening program

Make copies of this checklist (or download it from our website www.csiro.au/clip) and fill it out for the applicable exercises every day you do them. If there are beginner, intermediate and advanced levels for the exercise, make a note of which you do.

DATE:

warm-up (Y/N)   cool down (Y/N)

			set 1		set 2		set 3	
body region	muscle group	exercise	weight	reps	weight	reps	weight	reps
upper body	shoulders	one-arm front deltoid raise						
		lateral deltoid raise						
		overhead press						
	chest	push-up						
		chest fly with dumbbells						
	upper back	upright row						
		bent-over row						
	triceps	triceps dip						
		standing triceps kickback with dumbbells						
	biceps	biceps curl						
		hammer curl						
core	abdominals	half crunch						
		the plank						
	lower back	swim						
lower body	buttocks	lying buttocks bridge						
		glute kickback						
	upper leg	squat						
		lunge						
		step-up						
	lower leg	calf raise						

Appendix 3

CLIP eating plan checklist

Photocopy the checklist overleaf or download it from our website (www.csiro.au/clip) and fill it in each day. Here are some tips for filling in your own checklist.

- Fill in the checklist each day referring to pages 106–107 for units and quantities of each food type.
- Incorporate legumes into your lunch and dinner meals twice a week.
- Eat fish twice at lunch and twice at dinner each week.
- For extra cholesterol-lowering effect, choose 3 serves of plant-sterol-enriched foods each day.
- If you have eaten the foods listed in the amounts advised, simply write the food type in the box. For example:
  * low-fat milk or low-fat yoghurt in the dairy box
  * shaved turkey in the lunch protein box, or
  * wholegrain bread in the lunch carbohydrate box.
- If you have eaten the food, but have had more or less than advised, also write in the amount you ate. You will always need to do this for dinner protein and dinner carbohydrate, as these can vary depending on whether you choose Option 1 or Option 2. For example:
  * beef, 100 g in the dinner protein box
  * potato, 150 g in the dinner carbohydrate box
  * apple, 200 g in the fruit box
  * low-fat milk, 150 ml in the dairy box.

- If you have not eaten a food at all, simply put a cross in the box.
- Record the type and quantity of *all* other foods you have eaten (whether they are allowed or not) in the indulgence foods box, for example:
  * diet soft drink 1 can, 375 ml
  * dark chocolate, 25 g.

WEEK: DATE:	Monday	Tuesday	Wednesday	Thursday	Friday	Saturday	Sunday
dinner protein (fish twice a week)							
dinner carbohydrate							
lunch protein (fish twice a week)							
lunch carbohydrate							
high-soluble-fibre cereal							
low-fat dairy or soy alternative							
cheese (twice a week only)							
vegetables – salad or cooked							
fruit							
fats & oils							
nuts							
indulgence foods or alcohol							
other foods							
other foods							
other foods							
physical activity							

Appendix 4

CLIP maintenance plan checklist

Once you start on the maintenance plan, fill out this checklist each day. Include all foods, whether or not they are allowed as part of the plan.

WEEK: DATE:	Monday	Tuesday	Wednesday	Thursday	Friday	Saturday	Sunday
dinner protein (fish twice a week)							
dinner carbohydrate							
lunch protein (fish twice a week)							
lunch carbohydrate							
high-soluble-fibre cereal							
low-fat dairy or soy alternative							
cheese (twice a week only)							
vegetables – salad or cooked							
fruit							
fats & oils							
nuts							
indulgence foods or alcohol							
other foods							
other foods							
other foods							
500 kJ block							
500 kJ block							
500 kJ block							
500 kJ block							
physical activity							

500-kilojoule blocks

food or drink	500-kilojoule block	unit(s)
dried fruit – e.g. sultanas	60 grams (⅓ cup)	2 units fruit
fresh fruit salad	300 grams	2 units fruit
avocado	60 grams (¼ whole)	3 units fats and oils
seeds – sunflower, pumpkin, sesame	20 grams (1½ tablespoons)	1 unit nuts
dry-roasted, unsalted nuts	20 grams (approx. 15 assorted)	1 unit nuts
tahini paste	20 grams (1 tablespoon)	1 unit nuts
peanut butter	20 grams (3 teaspoons)	1 unit nuts
unsaturated oil – olive, canola, etc.	3 teaspoons	3 units fats and oils
bread – wholegrain, wholemeal, fruit	1 × 40-gram slice	1 unit carbohydrate
cooked pasta or rice	½ cup	1 unit carbohydrate
potato or sweet potato	150 grams	1 unit carbohydrate
low-fat milk, e.g. flavoured milk	250 millilitres (1 cup)	1 unit dairy
low-fat yoghurt or custard	200 grams (1 tub)	1 unit dairy
fromage frais	150 grams (1 tub)	1 unit dairy
plant protein foods – tofu, TVP, etc.	100 grams	1 unit protein
tinned beans or legumes (low-salt)	100 grams cooked	1 unit protein or 1 unit carbohydrate
low-fat ice-cream	70 grams (3 level scoops)	1 unit dairy
dark chocolate	25 grams	~1 unit indulgence
crisps – potato, chickpea, pita, soya, peas (cooked in canola or sunola oil)	1 × 21-gram packet	~1 unit indulgence
air-popped popcorn, no added salt	4 cups cooked	~1 unit indulgence
dried chickpeas	25 grams	~1 unit indulgence
wine	120 millilitres (1½ standard drinks)	~1 unit indulgence
beer	200 millilitres (1 standard drink)	~1 unit indulgence
spirits	50 millilitres (2 standard drinks)	~1 unit indulgence

Appendix 5

Vital statistics

Your cardiovascular health indicators

your vital statistics		Initial	6 weeks	1 year	2 years	3 years	4 years
blood cholesterol and triglycerides	total cholesterol						
	LDL cholesterol						
	HDL cholesterol						
	triglycerides						
blood pressure							
weight indicators	weight						
	BMI						
	waist circumference						
blood glucose							
exercise (minutes per day)							
smoking							
sleep (hours per night)							
stress (low, medium or high)							

Target cholesterol & triglyceride levels

	for the general population (mmol/L)*	for those at risk of CVD (mmol/L)**
triglycerides	less than 1.7	less than 1.5
total cholesterol	less than 5.2	less than 4.0
HDL cholesterol	males more than 1.0 females more than 1.3	more than 1.0
LDL cholesterol	less than 3.4	less than 2.5

* National Heart, Blood and Lung Institute recommendations
** Heart Foundation recommendations
Note that if you have been diagnosed with coronary heart disease or diabetes, you should aim for an LDL cholesterol level of less than 2.0.

Appendix 6

Shopping lists

This 'In the cupboard or fridge' list and the weekly shopping lists will provide you with all you need for the menu plans on pages 124–49. The quantities required will depend on how many people in your household are following CLIP. Copy the lists and fill in the quantities or download them with quantities from www.csiro.au/clip.

In the cupboard or fridge

almonds (blanched, flaked)
pine nuts
sesame seeds
unsalted, dry-roasted nuts
   (for daily snacks)
raisins
frozen peas
onions (brown, red)
garlic
ginger
eggs
low-fat sterol-enriched milk
low-fat flavoured yoghurt (can be
   sterol-enriched) or dairy desserts
sterol spread
wholegrain bread
wholegrain bread rolls
wholegrain crisp bread
high-soluble-fibre cereal
   (e.g. Guardian, Healthwise
   and/or Oatbrits)
unsweetened toasted muesli
unsweetened untoasted muesli
unflavoured, unsweetened instant oats
instant couscous
rice (arborio, basmati, long-grain)

soba noodles
balsamic vinegar
red-wine vinegar
rice-wine vinegar
flour (plain, plain wholemeal)
sugar (brown)
salt-reduced stock (beef, chicken,
   vegetable)
spices (black pepper; caraway seeds;
   cinnamon – ground, sticks; coriander –
   ground, seeds; dried chilli flakes,
   dukkah, fennel seeds, garam masala,
   ground cardamom, ground cloves,
   ground cumin, ground turmeric,
   low-salt curry powder, saffron
   threads, smoked paprika, sumac)
dried herbs (bay leaves, marjoram,
   mint, oregano, rosemary)
fish tinned in spring water (salmon,
   sardines, tuna)
honey
mustard (Dijon, wholegrain)
fat-free balsamic dressing
fat-free mayonnaise
fat-free salad dressing
apple sauce

cranberry sauce
low-salt soy sauce
oyster sauce
plum sauce
salt-reduced Worcestershire
   sauce
sweet chilli sauce
Tabasco sauce
curry paste (green, mild)
tom yum paste
salt-reduced tomato paste
hot mango chutney
salt-reduced tomato relish
gherkins
low-salt pickles
roasted red capsicums
   in a jar
tinned salt-reduced baked beans
canola oil
extra virgin olive oil
olive oil
sesame oil
canola oil spray
olive oil spray
tea and/or coffee
wine (red, white)

Week 1

fresh fruit (including lemons, orange)
avocado
broccoli
broccolini
capsicums (green, red, yellow)
carrots
celery
chillies (long green, long red)
cucumbers (Lebanese)
green beans
green vegetables (for steaming)
herbs (basil, coriander, flat-leaf parsley,
    rosemary, tarragon)
horseradish (or salt-reduced in jar)
mushrooms (mixed, portobello,
    Swiss brown)
pumpkin
salad leaves (baby cos, baby rocket,
    baby spinach, mixed leaves,
    rocket leaves)
snow peas
spring onions
tomatoes (including cherry, Roma)
zucchini
hot-smoked ocean trout
firm white fish (barramundi, gemfish
    or flathead)
salmon fillets
chicken thigh fillets
pork fillet and salt-reduced ham
roast beef, Scotch fillet and sirloin
    steaks
trimmed lamb shoulder
full-fat (or low-fat) cheddar
low-fat natural yoghurt
low-fat pizza cheese
Lebanese flatbreads
tinned salt-reduced three-bean mix
tinned salt-reduced chopped tomatoes
tinned salt-reduced sweet corn
marinated artichokes
raw or dry-roasted cashews

Week 2

fresh fruit (including lemons, limes,
    orange)
asparagus
broccoli
cabbage (green)
carrots
celery
chillies (long red)
fennel bulbs
green beans
herbs (coriander, dill, mint, sage,
    tarragon)
parsnips
potatoes
pumpkin (including butternut)
salad leaves (baby rocket, baby spinach,
    lettuce, mixed leaf, rocket, tabouli)
snow peas
spring onions
tomatoes (including cherry)
witlof
zucchini
firm white fish (barramundi, gemfish
    or flathead)
smoked salmon
salmon fillets
roast chicken (or beef), skinless thigh
    cutlets, skinless breast and smoked
    breast
pork loin cutlets and salt-reduced ham
roast beef (or chicken) and sirloin steaks
lamb shanks (on the bone, French-trimmed)
full-fat (or low-fat) cheddar
low-fat natural yoghurt
low-fat ricotta
Wholewheat Mountain Bread wraps
tinned salt-reduced cannellini beans
tinned salt-reduced lentils
marinated artichokes
low-fat hummus
apple juice

Week 3

fresh fruit (including lemons, lime)
asparagus
capsicums (red)
carrots (baby)
celery
chillies (long red)
cucumbers (Lebanese)
fennel bulbs
green beans
herbs (basil, coriander, flat-leaf parsley,
    mint, mixed, thyme)
mixed vegetables (for baking, salad)
potatoes (desiree or sweet, kipfler)
pumpkin (butternut)
salad leaves (baby spinach, lettuce,
    rocket)
snow peas
spring onions
tomatoes (including cherry, Roma)
zucchini
smoked trout
snapper fillets
mussels
prawns (uncooked)
chicken tenderloins and sliced breast
salt-reduced ham
rump and sirloin steaks and shaved
    roast beef
lamb backstraps and steaks
firm tofu
full-fat (or low-fat) cheddar
low-fat natural yoghurt
wholegrain pita bread
tinned salt-reduced cannellini beans
tinned salt-reduced chickpeas
tinned salt-reduced corn kernels
    (or fresh)
tinned salt-reduced chopped tomatoes
unsalted pistachios

Week 4

fresh fruit (including firm pears, lemons, limes, orange, pink grapefruit)
avocado
capsicums (red)
carrots
celery
chillies (long red)
cucumbers (including Lebanese)
fennel bulbs
green beans
herbs (basil, flat-leaf parsley, mixed, rosemary, thyme)
mixed vegetables (for salad, steaming, stir-frying)
mushrooms (small button)
potatoes (including chat)
salad leaves (baby cos, baby rocket, lettuce, mixed, watercress)
spring onions
tomatoes (including cherry)
witlof
zucchini
hot-smoked salmon
squid tubes
roast chicken (or beef), skinless drumsticks and smoked breast
shaved turkey
pork loin and shaved roast pork
roast beef (or chicken) and stewing beef
lamb steaks
low-salt feta
Swiss cheese
tinned salt-reduced three-bean mix
tinned salt-reduced lentils
tinned salt-reduced chopped tomatoes
marinated artichokes
dried cherries
can Guinness

Week 5

fresh fruit (including lemons, limes, orange)
broccolini
capsicums (red, yellow)
carrots
celery
chillies (long green, long red)
corn cobs
cucumbers (including Lebanese)
green beans
green vegetables (for salad)
herbs (basil, coriander, flat-leaf parsley, mint, Thai basil)
mixed vegetables (for salad, steaming)
potatoes (desiree)
pumpkin
salad leaves (baby spinach, coleslaw, lettuce, rocket, watercress)
snow peas
spring onions
tomatoes (including cherry)
zucchini
gemfish fillets
white fish fillets (perch, gemfish, cod or flathead)
shaved smoked chicken and skinless breasts
pork loin steaks and shaved roast pork
lean rump steak, Scotch fillet and shaved roast beef
lamb fillet
full-fat (or low-fat) cheddar
low-fat natural yoghurt
low-fat ricotta
tinned salt-reduced three-bean mix
tinned salt-reduced whole baby beetroot
tinned salt-reduced sweet corn
tinned salt-reduced chopped tomatoes
evaporated milk
low-fat hummus

Week 6

fresh fruit (including lemons, limes, mango)
alfalfa sprouts
avocado
bean sprouts
broccolini
capsicum (red)
chillies (long green, long red)
cucumbers (including Lebanese)
green beans
green vegetables (for salad)
herbs (basil, coriander, flat-leaf parsley, mint, mixed, Vietnamese mint)
leek
mixed vegetables (for salad)
mushrooms (mixed)
salad leaves (baby cos, baby spinach, butter lettuce, mixed, rocket)
snow pea sprouts
spring onions
tomatoes (including cherry)
smoked trout
king prawns (cooked, peeled and deveined with tails intact)
roast chicken and skinless thigh cutlets
shaved turkey
pork fillet and salt-reduced ham
minute and sirloin steaks
lean minced lamb
Sanitarium Vegie Delights mince (or TVP)
full-fat and/or low-fat cheddar
low-fat natural yoghurt
low-fat ricotta
tinned salt-reduced sliced beetroot
tinned salt-reduced corn kernels
salt-reduced tomato passata (puree)
burghul (cracked wheat)
raw or dry-roasted, unsalted cashews

Week 7

fresh fruit (including lemons, lime, orange)
avocado
capsicum (red)
carrots
celery
chilli (long red)
cucumber (Lebanese)
green beans
green vegetables (for salad)
herbs (coriander, flat-leaf parsley, mint, mixed, rosemary, thyme)
horseradish (or salt-reduced in jar)
mixed vegetables (for salad, steaming)
mushrooms (including small button)
potatoes (chat)
pumpkin
salad leaves (baby cos, baby rocket, baby spinach, mixed, rocket)
snow peas
spring onions
tomatoes (including cherry)
witlof
gemfish fillets
hot smoked salmon
smoked trout
chicken tenderloins and smoked breast
shaved turkey
salt-reduced ham and shaved roast pork
shaved roast beef and stewing beef
lamb steaks and lean minced lamb
low-fat cheddar
low-fat natural yoghurt
low-fat pizza cheese
wholemeal Lebanese flatbreads
tinned salt-reduced lentils
tinned salt-reduced white beans
salt-reduced tomato passata (puree)
salt-reduced tomato pasta sauce
marinated artichokes
fusilli pasta
can Guinness

Week 8

fresh fruit (including lemons, limes, orange)
avocado
broccoli
capsicums (red, yellow)
carrots
celery
chillies (long red)
green beans
herbs (basil, coriander, dill, flat-leaf parsley, mint, mixed, rosemary, tarragon)
mixed vegetables (for salad, steaming)
mushrooms
potatoes (desiree)
pumpkin (including butternut)
salad leaves (baby cos, baby spinach, mixed, rocket)
snow peas
spring onions
tomatoes (including cherry)
zucchini
salmon fillets and sliced smoked salmon
smoked trout
prawns (uncooked)
squid tubes
skinless chicken thigh cutlets and smoked breast
pork fillet and salt-reduced ham
sirloin steaks
lamb fillet
full-fat (or low-fat) cheddar
low-fat natural yoghurt
tinned salt-reduced cannellini beans

Week 9

fresh fruit (including lemons, lime)
avocado
cabbage (green)
carrots (baby)
celery
cucumber
fennel bulbs
green beans
green vegetables (for salad)
herbs (basil, coriander, flat-leaf parsley, mint, sage, thyme)
leek
mixed vegetables (for baking, steaming)
parsnips
potatoes (kipfler)
pumpkin (butternut)
salad leaves (baby rocket, butter lettuce, lettuce, mixed)
snow peas
spring onions
tomatoes
witlof
salmon fillets
snapper fillets
sliced chicken breast and smoked breast
pork loin, pork loin cutlets and salt-reduced ham
shaved roast beef
lamb backstraps
firm tofu
full-fat and/or low-fat cheddar
low-fat natural yoghurt
low-fat ricotta
wholemeal pita bread
tinned salt-reduced cannellini beans
tinned salt-reduced lentils
tinned salt-reduced three-bean mix
tinned salt-reduced chopped tomatoes
marinated artichokes
dried cherries
unsalted pistachios
apple juice

Week 10

fresh fruit (including lemons, limes)
avocado
broccolini
capsicums (red)
carrots
celery
chilli (long green)
cucumbers
green beans
herbs (basil, coriander, flat-leaf parsley, mint, tarragon)
horseradish (or salt-reduced in jar)
mixed vegetables (for salad)
mushrooms (mixed, portobello)
pumpkin
salad leaves (mixed, watercress, rocket)
spring onions
tomatoes (including cherry)
zucchini
salmon fillets
white fish fillets (perch, gemfish, cod or flathead)
prawns (uncooked)
roast chicken and skinless breasts
shaved turkey
pork fillet and shaved roast pork
lean roast beef and sirloin steaks
lamb cutlets and shanks (on the bone, French-trimmed)
full-fat (or low-fat) cheddar
low-salt feta
low-fat natural yoghurt
tinned salt-reduced cannellini beans
tinned salt-reduced three-bean mix
tinned salt-reduced whole baby beetroot
raw or dry-roasted cashews

Week 11

fresh fruit (including lemons, lime, orange)
asparagus
avocado
capsicums (red, yellow)
carrots
celery
chillies (long red)
cucumbers (including Lebanese)
fennel bulbs
green beans
herbs (basil, coriander, flat-leaf parsley, mint, rosemary)
mixed vegetables (for steaming)
pumpkin (butternut)
salad leaves (baby spinach, coleslaw, mixed, rocket, watercress)
snow peas
spring onions
tomatoes (including cherry, Roma)
zucchini
salmon fillets
shaved smoked chicken and skinless drumsticks
pork loin steaks and shaved roast pork
Scotch fillet and shaved roast beef
trimmed lamb shoulder
full-fat (or low-fat) cheddar
low-salt feta
low-fat natural yoghurt
tinned salt-reduced lentils
tinned salt-reduced three-bean mix
tinned salt-reduced chopped tomatoes
low-fat hummus

Week 12

fresh fruit (including lemons, limes, mango)
alfalfa sprouts
avocado
bean sprouts
broccoli
broccolini
capsicum (red)
celery
chillies (long green, long red)
cucumbers (Lebanese)
green beans
herbs (basil, coriander, flat-leaf parsley, lemon thyme, mint, Thai basil, Vietnamese mint)
mixed vegetables (for salad)
potatoes (desiree)
salad leaves (baby spinach, butter, lettuce, lettuce, mixed, rocket, tabouli)
snow pea sprouts
spring onions
sweet corn (kernels – fresh or tinned)
tomatoes (including cherry, Roma)
zucchini
smoked trout
cooked crabmeat
king prawns (cooked)
chicken thigh fillets and thigh cutlets
shaved turkey
salt-reduced ham
roast beef and rump steak
lamb (for kebabs) and lamb cutlets
Sanitarium Vegie Delights Mince (or TVP)
full-fat (or low-fat) cheddar
low-fat natural yoghurt
low-fat ricotta
wholemeal Mountain Bread wraps
tinned salt-reduced chopped tomatoes
dried linguine
burghul (cracked wheat)
low-fat hummus

Vegetarian

fresh fruit (including lemons, limes, orange)
capsicum (red)
carrots (including baby)
celery
chillies (long red)
cucumbers (including Lebanese)
eggplant
fennel bulbs
green vegetables (for salad)
herbs (basil, coriander, flat-leaf parsley, mint)
leek
mixed vegetables (for salad, stir-frying)
pumpkin
salad leaves (baby spinach, butter lettuce, mixed, watercress)
snow peas
spring onions
sweet potato
tomatoes (including cherry)
firm tofu
Sanitarium Vegie Delights Mince (or TVP)
low-fat cheddar
low-fat natural yoghurt
low-fat pizza cheese
low-fat ricotta
tinned salt-reduced cannellini beans
tinned salt-reduced lentils
tinned salt-reduced chopped tomatoes
salt-reduced tomato passata (puree)
fresh lasagne sheets
filo pastry
unsalted pistachios

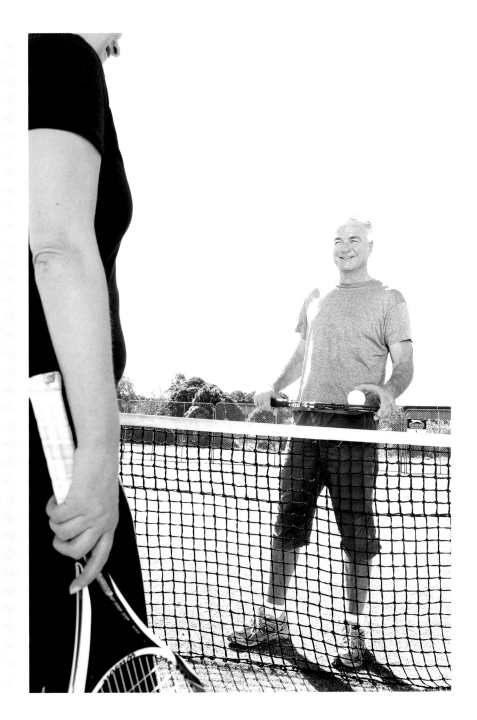

Index

A

abdominal exercises 84–5
abdominal fat
  and blood pressure 17
  and cardiovascular disease 17
  and exercise 34
  effect of gender 17
  and osteoarthritis 17
  and sleep apnoea 17
  and stroke 17
  and type 2 diabetes 17
  see also waist circumference
ACE inhibitors 30
activity levels 19
aerobic exercise 4, 29, 34–5, 36, 60,
  61, 68–72, 255–60
aerobic fitness 72, 255–7
aerobic walking 29, 61, 68–72
ALA (alpha-linolenic acid) 95
alcohol
  abuse and depression 44, 46
  and blood pressure 27, 29
  and cardiovascular health 25, 26,
    27, 29, 51, 98, 119
  and cholesterol 98
  on CLIP 29, 98, 106, 113, 121
  cutting down 27, 51, 55
  when eating out 55, 113
  and erectile dysfunction 39
  and HDL cholesterol 25
  kilojoule content 20, 98, 264
  recommended intake 29, 98
  and sleep 50
  standard drink 98
almonds
  . . . on CLIP 96, 111, 116, 117
  apple & almond strudel 245
  beetroot & almond salad 189
  sumac-roasted chicken with beetroot
    & almond salad 189
angina 1, 22, 30, 40, 47
angiotensin-receptor blockers 30
apple & almond strudel 245
arteries
  and abdominal fat 17
  and cholesterol 22, 23

definition 1
effect of CLIP 3
elasticity 1
inflammation 1, 23
narrowing 1, 31
arthritis and exercise 68
artichoke
  creamy artichoke dip 172
  pizza with tomato, artichoke &
    mushrooms 163
artificial sweeteners 105
asparagus
  beetroot & asparagus salad 199
  chargrilled asparagus 202
asthma 30
atherosclerosis
  and the brain 2
  and blood clots 2, 47
  and blood pressure 1
  and cardiovascular disease 47
  causes 1, 31
  and cholesterol 1
  and erectile dysfunction 2, 40
  and exercise 2
  and heart attack 2
  and long-chain omega-3 fatty
    acids 93
  risk factors 1
  and smoking 1
  and stress 47
  and stroke 2
avocado
  . . . fat content 24
  . . . heart-protective food 108, 264
  . . . oil 99
  avocado & corn dip 172
  avocado salad with tahini dressing
    203
  cucumber & avocado sushi 250
  smoked trout & avocado on rye 250

B

baked beans
  recipe 206
  tinned 28, 97, 103
baked snapper fillets with lemon &

thyme potatoes 213
banana & blueberry smoothie 155
barbecue for 6 200–3
barbecued sirloin with mustard crust &
  portobello mushrooms 183
beef
  . . . on CLIP 106, 117
  barbecued sirloin with mustard crust
    & portobello mushrooms 183
  beef & Guinness casserole 232
  chargrilled beef with zucchini, pine
    nuts & spinach 178
  chargrilled steak sandwiches with
    tomato relish 232
  Thai beef kebabs 192
beetroot
  beetroot & asparagus salad 199
  beetroot & almond salad 189
bent-over row 80
beta blockers 30, 71
biceps
  curl 82
  exercises 82–3
blocks (500 kJ)
  adding to maintenance plan 109,
    120–1
  examples 121, 264
blood clots
  and atherosclerosis 2
  and long-chain omega-3 fatty
    acids 93
  and stress 47
blood glucose
  as cardiovascular disease risk factor
    12, 31
  effects of 31
  and erectile dysfunction 41
  and exercise 34
  glucose intolerance 2, 12
  and HDL cholesterol 31
  and heart attack 33
  measurement 12
  and pre-diabetes 12
  and sexual problems 39
  and sleep 49
  and stress 42

and triglycerides 31
and type 2 diabetes 12, 31–3
blood pressure
    and abdominal fat 17
    and atherosclerosis 1
    and cardiovascular disease 2, 13,
        47, 48
    and cholesterol 10, 265
    definition 11, 27
    diastolic blood pressure 11
    effect of CLIP 3
    and erectile dysfunction 41
    and exercise 27, 29, 34, 59
    family history 27
    and heart attack 2, 11, 27
    and kidney disease 11, 27
    and lifestyle 27
    lowering 27–8
    measurement 11, 27
    medication 29, 30
    and long-chain omega-3 fatty
        acids 93
    recommended levels 11, 27, 265
    and salt intake 27
    and sleep 49, 50
    and sleep apnoea 13, 49
    and stress 29, 42, 47, 48
    and stroke 2, 11, 27
    systolic blood pressure 11
    and triglycerides 10, 265
    and weight loss 27
blood sugar *see* blood glucose
BMI
    and cardiovascular disease 11
    and ethnic origin 10
    measurement 10, 18
    and obesity 10
body mass index *see* BMI
braised pork with dried cherries 190
bread
    . . . carbohydrate content 31
    king prawns with crusty bread 202
    pita bread, tomato & tuna salad 164
    pita crisps 173
    . . . wholegrain 97, 108
brunches for 4 154–5
bruschetta
    bruschetta with hummus, roasted
        vegetables & basil 160
    tomato bruschetta 251
buckwheat noodles 215

buttermilk panna cotta 203
buttocks exercises 86

C
calcium 95, 111, 118
calcium-channel blockers 30
calf raise 88
calves stretch 62
cancer 1, 44, 252
capsicums
    capsicum & fennel salad 183
    chargrilled lamb fillets with
        pepperonata 197
    crudités 173
    marinated fish skewers with
        capsicum & fennel salad 183
    spicy roasted capsicum dip 172
carbohydrate blockers 32
carbohydrates 252
    on CLIP 103, 106, 113, 117
    complex 31
    effect on triglyceride levels 26
    glucose 31–3
    refined 26, 97, 99
    sugar 52
    see also wholegrain cereals
cardiovascular disease (CVD)
    252
    and alcohol 98
    and blood pressure 2, 13, 47
    and cholesterol 2, 13, 22, 48
    and CLIP 3
    and diet 1
    and exercise 2, 12, 34–5, 59, 70
    and family history 2, 9
    and genetic make-up 2
    lifestyle as prevention 2
    motivation for treatment 51–5
    New Zealand Heart Disease Risk
        Calculator 10
    and obesity 10
    premature heart disease 2
    protective foods 2–3, 119
    risk factors 9–13, 22, 120, 265
    and shorter-chain omega-3 fatty
        acids 111–12
    and sleep 50
    and sleep apnoea 49
    and smoking 2, 13, 48
    and stress 47–8
    and triglycerides 25

and type 2 diabetes 2, 10, 22
and vegetarians 110, 112
warning signs 9–13, 17
cardiovascular exercise 61, 68
carrots
    carrot & ginger soup 168
    crudités 173
    roasted carrot, tofu & fennel
        salad 160
    slow-cooked lamb shanks with
        beans, carrots & spring
        onions 228
    spicy carrot & yoghurt dip 173
cereals 116
    carbohydrate content 31
    see also wholegrain cereals
champagne cocktail 251
chargrilled asparagus 202
chargrilled beef with zucchini, pine
    nuts & spinach 178
chargrilled lamb fillets with
    pepperonata 197
chargrilled salmon with lentils, spinach
    & yoghurt 211
chargrilled squid salad 179
chargrilled steak sandwiches with
    tomato relish 232
checklists 21, 105, 258–63
cheese 106, 118
chest exercises 78–9
chest fly with dumbbells 79
chest stretch 66
chicken
    . . . and blood pressure 29
    . . . on CLIP 103, 106, 117
    . . . as protein source 99
    . . . salt content 28
    chicken & vegetable paella 220
    chicken dumpling & noodle soup
        with greens 226
    chicken dumplings 226
    chicken, snow pea & pumpkin
        salad 164
    harissa chicken with tabouli 223
    sesame chicken with soba noodles &
        plum sauce 224
    smoked chicken & pesto
        sandwiches 250
    smoked chicken, green bean & lentil
        salad with sesame seeds 220
    spiced chicken casserole 189

sticky chicken drumsticks 184
sumac-roasted chicken with beetroot
    & almond salad 189
chickpeas
    . . . tinned 97
    tabouli & chickpea salad 203
    thyme & lemon lamb cutlets with
        zucchini & chickpea salad 230
    zucchini & chickpea salad 230
chocolate
    . . . on CLIP 107, 119
    . . . health benefits 119
    chocolate pots 242
    hot chocolate puddings 237
cholesterol
    and angina 22
    and artery health 1
    and atherosclerosis 1
    and cardiovascular disease 2, 9–10,
        13
    cholesterol status 9
    effect of CLIP 3, 115
    definition 22, 252
    and eggs 25, 118
    and erectile dysfunction 41
    functions 22
    and heart attack 2
    medications 3, 26
    effect of plant sterols 25, 98, 254
    recommended levels 22, 23, 265
    and saturated fat 119
    and sexual problems 39
    and sleep 50
    and stroke 2, 22
    total cholesterol 9, 252, 265
    and weight loss 108–9
    see also HDL ('good') cholesterol, LDL
        ('bad') cholesterol
cholesterol-lowering medications 3, 26
CLIP 2–3, 113–19, 253
    effect on arteries 3
    basic plan 106–7, 108–9
    blocks (500 kJ) 109, 120–1, 264
    effect on blood pressure 3
    carbohydrate 106, 113, 117
    and cardiovascular health 93, 265
    checklists 21, 105, 258–63
    cheese 106, 118
    effect on cholesterol 3, 93, 103, 115
    clinical trials 3
    daily food allowance 104, 106–7

eating out on 20–1, 55, 113–14
eating plan 93, 103–21
and erectile dysfunction 41
and exercise 34–8, 121
exercise program 35, 57–89
fats 107
and fibre 95
and fish 106, 261
fruit 107, 117
heart-protective foods 108–9,
    120–1, 119, 264
indulgence foods 107
kilojoule levels 104, 108–9
legumes 106, 117, 261
low-fat dairy foods 95, 104, 106,
    116–17
maintenance plan 108, 109, 120–1
menu plans 122–49
nuts 96, 107, 117
oils 107, 116
Option 1 dinners 103, 109, 115,
    116, 175–97, 261
Option 2 dinners 103, 109, 115,
    205–33, 261
plant-sterol-enriched foods in 25,
    104, 106, 107, 116
protein 103, 106, 113, 117, 118
and salt intake 104
shopping lists 266–9
tailoring to your needs 3
ten super CLIP foods 93–9, 104
and triglycerides 3, 97, 103
vegetables 107, 113, 114, 117
for vegetarians 110–12
and weight loss 2, 3, 18, 103, 108–9
wholegrain cereals 106
cocktail party for 8 248–51
comfort food 47
Comprehensive Lifestyle Program
    see CLIP
condiments on Free List 105
cool-down after exercise 61
core exercises 74, 84–5
couscous 216
creamy artichoke dip 172
crudités 173
cucumber
    cucumber & avocado sushi 250
    prawn & cucumber salad with
        mango 180
cumin yoghurt 178

curried sweet potato cakes 208
CVD see cardiovascular disease

D
dairy foods see low-fat dairy foods
depression 42–8
    and blood-pressure medication 30
    and cardiovascular disease 13,
        42, 48
    and exercise 34
    and overeating 53
    seeking help 47
    and sleep 49
    and stress 42–8, 53, 55
    symptoms 13, 47
desserts 237, 239–47
diabetes see pre-diabetes; type 2
    diabetes
dinner
    for 4 234–7
    Option 1 recipes 175–97
    Option 2 recipes 205–33
dips
    . . . when eating out on CLIP 114
    avocado & corn 172
    creamy artichoke 172
    roasted eggplant 172
    spicy carrot & yoghurt 173
    spicy roasted capsicum 172
diuretics 30
dressings
    . . . when eating out on CLIP 113
    herb aïoli 158
    horseradish 158
    lemon yoghurt 163, 216
    minted chilli 184
    for prawn & cucumber salad 180
    sweet chilli mayonnaise 224
    tahini 203
drinks
    . . . on Free List 105
    banana & blueberry smoothie 155
    champagne cocktail 251
    mocktail Moscow mule 202
    pomegranate fizz 251
    ruby grapefruit, blood orange &
        minted pineapple juice 154
dukkah-crusted salmon with
    couscous 216
dumbbells 73, 74, 75–6

E

eating out on CLIP 20–1, 55, 113–14
eggplant
    roasted eggplant dip 172
eggs
    and blood pressure 29
    and cholesterol 25, 118
    and long-chain omega-3 fatty acids
        118–19
    recommended intake 25, 106, 118
energy needs *see* kilojoule needs
erectile dysfunction (ED) 40–1
    and atherosclerosis 2, 40
    and blood glucose 41
    and blood pressure 41
    and blood-pressure medication 30
    and cardiovascular disease 13, 39, 40
    and cholesterol 41
    and CLIP 41
    and depression 40
    and diet 41
    and exercise 41
    and sleep apnoea 13, 49
    treatment 41
    and type 2 diabetes 39, 40
    and weight loss 41
exercise
    and atherosclerosis 12
    and blood pressure 27, 29, 59
    and cardiovascular disease 2, 12, 34,
        48, 59, 70
    and cholesterol 34
    diary 60, 76, 261
    with dumbbells 73, 74, 75–6
    for heart health 34–8
    at home 37
    in leisure time 37
    and maintenance 121
    motivation for 51–5, 59–60
    and obesity 59
    recommendations 36–8
    reps 74
    safety 75–6
    sets 74
    sex 39
    and sleep 49
    and smoking 59
    and stroke 59
    and tiredness 37
    when travelling 38
    and triglycerides 32, 34

and type 2 diabetes 32, 59, 70
and weight 59
at work 37
see also aerobic exercise
exercise program
    aerobic walking program 68–72,
        259
    checklists 60, 258–60
    CLIP 57–89
    cool-down 61
    muscle-strengthening program 60,
        61, 73–89, 260
    planning 38
    stretching 61–7
    warm-up 61
ezetimibe 26

F

familial hypercholesterolaemia 2, 9, 23
fast food 52
fats 253
    on CLIP 107
    healthy 25
    saturated 23–4, 25, 41, 99, 118,
        119, 253
    trans 24–5, 119, 253
    unsaturated 41, 96, 112, 116, 119,
        253
    see also oils
fennel
    capsicum & fennel salad 183
    fennel & rosemary pork with wilted
        spinach & roast potatoes 226
    marinated fish skewers with
        capsicum & fennel salad 183
    roasted carrot, tofu & fennel salad 160
fibrates 26
fibre *see* insoluble fibre; soluble fibre
fish
    . . . and blood pressure 29
    . . . on CLIP 29, 94, 103, 106,
        114, 117
    . . . heart-protective food 108
    . . . mercury levels 95
    . . . and omega-3 fatty acids 29,
        93–5, 254
    . . . as protein source 99
    . . . salt content 28, 117
    . . . suggested intake 94
    . . . tinned 28, 104, 111, 106, 117
    baked snapper fillets with lemon

        & thyme potatoes 213
    chargrilled salmon with lentils,
        spinach & yoghurt 211
    dukkah-crusted salmon with
        couscous 216
    fish & vegetable skewers 179
    fish chowder 213
    hot-smoked salmon, watercress
        & pink grapefruit salad 184
    pita bread, tomato & tuna
        salad 164
    roasted gemfish with saffron &
        cardamom pumpkin 186
    roasted salmon salad with minted
        chilli dressing 186
    smoked trout & avocado on
        rye 250
    smoked trout salad with orange,
        green beans & horseradish 158
    steamed ocean trout with buckwheat
        noodles 215
    Thai green fish curry 211
    tuna, corn & coriander patties 224
    tuna pasta bake 215
Free List 105
freshly shucked oysters 250
frittata
    pea, leek & mint frittata 154
fruit
    and blood pressure 28
    carbohydrate content 31
    on CLIP 3, 29, 107, 117
    and erectile dysfunction 41
    fibre content 20, 95
    heart-protective food 108
    recommended intake 29
    salt content 28
    and triglycerides 97
    water content 20
    and weight loss 52
    see also particular fruits
functional foods 3, 99

G

glitazones 32
glucose *see* blood glucose
glute kickback 86
gout 30
grapefruit
    hot-smoked salmon, watercress &
        pink grapefruit salad 184

ruby grapefruit, blood orange & minted pineapple juice 154
green beans
    oregano & lemon lamb with green beans & butternut pumpkin 194
    smoked trout salad with orange, green beans & horseradish 158
    stir-fried pork with green beans & mixed mushrooms 190
green chilli sauce 192
green vegie salad 199

H

half crunch 84
hammer curl 83
hamstrings stretch 63
harissa
    paste 223
    harissa chicken with tabouli 223
HDL ('good') cholesterol 252, 265
    and blood glucose 31
    effect of gender 25
    and heart attack 2
    how to increase 25
    protective role 22, 25
    as risk factor for cardiovascular disease 9–10
    and stroke 2
    during weight loss 24, 25
heart attack
    and atherosclerosis 2
    and blood glucose 33
    and ethnic background 2
    and exercise 34
    and long-chain omega-3 fatty acids 93
    medication 30
    risk factors 2, 9–13, 22, 27, 44, 47
    and sleep apnoea 49
heart disease *see* cardiovascular disease
heart failure 30
Heart Foundation 23, 25, 28, 34, 47–8, 97, 111, 112, 119
heart-protective foods 108–9, 119, 120–1, 264
heart rate 69–71, 72, 256
herb aïoli 158
high-density lipoprotein cholesterol *see* HDL ('good') cholesterol
horseradish dressing 158
hot & sour pumpkin soup 168
hot chocolate puddings 237

hot smoked salmon, watercress & pink grapefruit salad 184
hypertension 44, 47, 49

I

Indian pork curry with minted yoghurt & basmati rice 228
indulgence foods 107
inner thighs stretch 64
insoluble fibre 20, 97, 253
insulin 31–3, 34, 41, 254

J

jogging 29, 36, 61, 68, 72

K

kidney disease
    effect of blood glucose 31
    effect of blood pressure 11, 27
    and blood-pressure medication 30
    and heart attack 2
    and long-chain omega-3 fatty acids 94
    and stroke 2
    and type 2 diabetes 32
kilojoule needs
    calculating 19, 108
    levels for CLIP 108–9
    for maintenance 108, 109, 120–1
    for weight loss 18, 52
king prawns with crusty bread 202

L

lamb
    . . . on CLIP 106, 117
    chargrilled lamb fillets with pepperonata 197
    lamb & spinach meatballs with spicy tomato sauce 197
    oregano & lemon lamb with green beans & butternut pumpkin 194
    roast lamb with sweet potato 236
    slow-cooked lamb shanks with beans, carrots & spring onions 228
    thyme & lemon lamb cutlets with zucchini & chickpea salad 230
    winter lamb casserole 194
lateral deltoid raise 77
LDL ('bad') cholesterol 2, 24, 252, 265
    effect of CLIP 3, 23
    and full-fat dairy foods 95

and eggs 25
and exercise 34
and heart attack 2
and nuts 96
and plant sterols 98
recommended levels 23
as risk factor for cardiovascular disease 9–10, 22, 119
and shellfish 25
and soy products 99
and stroke 2
triggers 23
legumes 96–7, 254
    and blood pressure 29
    on CLIP 97, 103, 117
    and erectile dysfunction 41
    fibre content 95, 96
    protein content 117
    tinned 28, 97
    types 97
    see also particular legumes
lemons
    baked snapper fillets with lemon & thyme potatoes 213
    lemon vinaigrette 164, 184
    lemon yoghurt dressing 163, 216
    oregano & lemon lamb with green beans & butternut pumpkin 194
    prawn & salmon risotto with lemon & zucchini 218
    thyme & lemon lamb cutlets with zucchini & chickpea salad 230
    wholemeal lemon crepes with raspberries 246
lentils
    . . . tinned 97, 103
    chargrilled salmon with lentils, spinach & yoghurt 211
linguine with crab, lime & coriander 218
long-chain omega-3 fatty acids 254
    and blood pressure 29, 93
    in eggs 25, 118–19
    in fish 29, 93–5
    health benefits 93–4
    sources 93, 94–5
    suggested intake 94
    for vegetarians 111–12, 118–19
low-density lipoprotein cholesterol *see* LDL ('bad') cholesterol
low-fat dairy foods 95, 261

and blood pressure 29
on CLIP 95, 104, 106, 116–17
heart-protective food 108
lower-back exercise 85
lower-body exercises 74, 86–9
lower-body stretches 62–4
lower-leg exercises 88–9
lunches 157–65
lunge 87
lying buttocks bridge 86

M

maintenance plan 108, 109, 120–1
margarine
on CLIP 95, 104, 119
plant-sterol-enriched 3, 104, 108, 116, 119
and trans fats 24, 119
marinated fish skewers with capsicum & fennel salad 183
meat *see* beef; chicken; fish; lamb; pork; red meat
medication 120
for blood pressure 29, 30
for cholesterol 3, 26
and erectile dysfunction 40
meditation 29, 46
menu plans 122–49
metformin 32
milk
on CLIP 104, 116
flavoured 20
full-fat 95
plant-sterol-enriched 3, 104
minted chilli dressing 186
mocktail Moscow mule 202
monounsaturated fats 96, 116, 253
motivation
to exercise 51–5, 59–60
for weight loss 51–5
muscle groups 74
muscle-strengthening program 4, 29, 34–5, 60, 61, 73–89, 260
mushrooms
barbecued sirloin with mustard crust & portobello mushrooms 183
pizza with tomato, artichoke & mushrooms 163
stir-fried pork with green beans & mixed mushrooms 190
mustard crust (for coating steak) 183

N

negative self-talk 43, 45
New Zealand Heart Disease Risk Calculator 10
noodles
buckwheat noodles 215
sesame chicken with soba noodles & plum sauce 224
steamed ocean trout with buckwheat noodles 215
nuts 95–6
and blood pressure 29
and cardiovascular disease 96
on CLIP 2, 95–6, 99, 105, 107, 108, 109, 117, 121
in cooking 105
and erectile dysfunction 41
fat content 2, 24, 96, 99, 116
fibre content 96
kilojoule content 96, 264
and LDL cholesterol 96
and plant sterols 96, 98
protein content 95
recommended intake 96
salt content 28
for vegetarians 110, 111
see also particular nuts

O

oats 2, 95, 106, 108
obesity 2, 10, 44, 59
oils 99, 107, 116
omega-3 fatty acids *see* long-chain omega-3 fatty acids; shorter-chain omega-3 fatty acids
one-arm front deltoid raise 77
Option 1 dinners 103, 109, 115, 116, 175–97, 261
Option 2 dinners 103, 109, 115, 205–33, 261
oranges
ruby grapefruit, blood orange & minted pineapple juice 154
papaya & strawberry fruit plate with passionfruit & orange 246
smoked trout salad with orange, green beans & horseradish 158
oregano & lemon lamb with green beans & butternut pumpkin 194
osteoarthritis 1, 13
overhead press 78

P

pancreas 31–3
papaya & strawberry fruit plate with passionfruit & orange 246
pasta
. . . carbohydrate content 31
. . . wholegrain 97
linguine with crab, lime & coriander 218
tuna pasta bake 215
pea, leek & mint frittata 154
physical activity *see* exercise
pioglitazone 32
pita bread, tomato & tuna salad 164
pita crisps 173
pizza with tomato, artichoke & mushrooms 163
plank, the 85
plant sterols 98–99, 254
action 25
and cholesterol 25, 98
in CLIP 25, 99, 104, 106, 107, 116, 261
definition 25
in enriched margarine 3, 99, 107, 116, 119
in enriched milk 3, 99, 106
in enriched yoghurt 99, 106
in functional foods 3
sources 98
for vegetarians 112
plums
plum & hazelnut crumble 242
poached stone fruit with yoghurt 240
poached stone fruit with yoghurt 240
polyunsaturated fats 41, 96, 112, 116, 253
pomegranate fizz 251
pork
. . . and blood pressure 29
. . . on CLIP 103, 106, 117
braised pork with dried cherries 190
fennel & rosemary pork with wilted spinach & roast potatoes 226
Indian pork curry with minted yoghurt & basmati rice 228
marinated fish skewers with capsicum & fennel salad 183

pork cutlets with cabbage, parsnips
& raisins 192
salt content 28
stir-fried pork with green beans &
mixed mushrooms 190
portion control 20–1, 52
positive self-talk 45
potato
baked snapper fillets with lemon &
thyme potatoes 213
fennel & rosemary pork with wilted
spinach & roast potatoes 226
sweet corn & potato rösti 155
see also sweet potato
prawns
king prawns with crusty bread 202
prawn & cucumber salad with
mango 180
prawn & salmon risotto with lemon
& zucchini 218
prawn & tomato soup with mussels 180
pre-diabetes 12
premature heart disease 2
processed food 27
protein-rich foods 25, 29, 99, 118, 254
animal sources 99, 117
and blood pressure 29
on CLIP 29, 103, 106, 113, 117
functions 99
and heart health 99, 109
and hunger 20
low-fat dairy 95
nuts 95
soy products 97, 99, 110, 112
for vegetarians 110, 112
pumpkin
chicken, snow pea & pumpkin salad 164
hot & sour pumpkin soup 168
oregano & lemon lamb with green
beans & butternut pumpkin 194
pumpkin salad 199
roasted gemfish with saffron &
cardamom pumpkin 186
push-up 78–9

Q

quadriceps stretch 63

R

raspberry jelly with custard 240
red meat 29

on CLIP 103
as protein source 99
salt content 28
see also beef; lamb
resistance training see muscle-
strengthening program
rice
Indian pork curry with minted
yoghurt & basmati rice 228
prawn & salmon risotto with lemon
& zucchini 218
roast lamb with sweet potato 236
roasted carrot, tofu & fennel salad 160
roasted eggplant dip 172
roasted gemfish with saffron &
cardamom pumpkin 186
roasted salmon salad with minted chilli
dressing 186
rosiglitazone 32
ruby grapefruit, blood orange & minted
pineapple juice 154

S

salad suggestions 199
salads
avocado salad with tahini dressing
203
beetroot & almond salad 189
beetroot & asparagus salad 199
capsicum & fennel salad 183
chargrilled squid salad 179
chicken, snow pea & pumpkin salad
164
green vegie salad 199
hot smoked salmon, watercress &
pink grapefruit salad 184
pita bread, tomato & tuna salad 164
prawn & cucumber salad with
mango 180
pumpkin salad 199
roasted carrot, tofu & fennel salad
160
roasted salmon salad with minted
chilli dressing 186
sesame spinach salad 199
smoked chicken, green bean & lentil
salad with sesame seeds 220
smoked trout salad with orange,
green beans & horseradish 158
suggestions 199
tabouli & chickpea salad 203

tomato & herb salad 199
zucchini & chickpea salad 230
salmon 28; see also fish
salt
alternative flavours 28
and blood pressure 27–8
on CLIP 104, 114, 117
high-salt foods 28, 118
low-salt foods 28
in processed foods 27
recommended intake 28
reducing intake 27–8
sandwich suggestions 198
saturated fats 23–4, 25, 41, 95, 96, 99,
118, 119, 253
seafood
. . . cholesterol content 25
chargrilled squid salad 179
freshly shucked oysters 250
king prawns with crusty bread 202
linguine with crab, lime & coriander
218
prawn & cucumber salad with
mango 180
prawn & salmon risotto with lemon
& zucchini 218
prawn & tomato soup with mussels
180
sedentary behaviour 35, 36, 37
seeds 99
sesame seeds 117
sesame chicken with soba noodles &
plum sauce 224
sesame spinach salad 199
sex and weight loss 39
sexual problems 13, 39–41
see also erectile dysfunction
shopping lists 266–9
shorter-chain omega-3 fatty acids 93,
94, 95, 96, 110, 111–12, 117
shoulder exercises 77–8
shoulder stretches 65
sides stretch 67
sleep 49–50
and blood glucose 49
and blood pressure 49, 50
and cardiovascular disease 50
and cholesterol 50
and depression 13, 49
and erectile dysfunction 39
and exercise 49

and insulin 49
and stress 46–7
tips for good sleep 50
and type 2 diabetes 49
and weight 49, 50
sleep apnoea 49–50
and abdominal fat 17
and cardiovascular disease 49
diagnosis 49–50
and exercise 49
and gender 49
risks of 13, 49
and snoring 12–13, 49
symptoms 12–13, 50
and weight 49
slow-cooked lamb shanks with beans,
carrots & spring onions 228
smoked chicken & pesto sandwiches
250
smoked chicken, green bean & lentil
salad with sesame seeds 220
smoked trout
smoked trout & avocado on rye
250
smoked trout salad with orange,
green beans & horseradish 158
smoking
effect on artery health 12
and atherosclerosis 1
and blood clots 12
and cardiovascular disease 2, 12, 13,
39, 48
effect on cholesterol levels 10
and erectile dysfunction 39
and exercise 59
snacks 52, 55, 122–49, 167–9
snoring 12–13, 49
soluble fibre 2, 95, 254
and cholesterol 20, 95
on CLIP 95
sources 2, 95
soup
carrot & ginger soup 168
chicken dumpling & noodle soup
with greens 226
hot & sour pumpkin soup 168
prawn & tomato soup with mussels
180
zucchini & feta soup 236
soy products
on CLIP 103, 116

fibre content 95
and LDL cholesterol 99
and shorter-chain omega-3 fatty
acids 111
textured vegetable protein 112
for vegetarians 110, 112
spiced chicken casserole 189
spicy carrot & yoghurt dip 173
spicy roasted capsicum dip 172
spinach
chargrilled beef with zucchini, pine
nuts & spinach 178
chargrilled salmon with lentils,
spinach & yoghurt 211
fennel & rosemary pork with wilted
spinach & roast potatoes 226
lamb & spinach meatballs with spicy
tomato sauce 197
sesame spinach salad 199
smoked chicken, green bean & lentil
salad with sesame seeds 220
squat 87
standard drinks 98
standing triceps kickback with
dumbbells 82
statins 3, 26
steamed ocean trout with buckwheat
noodles 215
step-up 88
sticky chicken drumsticks 184
stir-fried pork with green beans &
mixed mushrooms 190
strawberry ice-cream terrine 245
strength-training exercise see muscle-
strengthening program
stress 42–8
and blood glucose 42
and blood pressure 29, 42
and cardiovascular disease 13, 42,
43, 47–8
causes 42–3
and depression 42–8, 53
and diet 46–7
and erectile dysfunction 39
and exercise 46
effect on health 44
management 44–8, 53–5
and meditation 46
pressures 43
and sleep 46–7
stressors 43

symptoms 43–4, 46
types 43
stretching exercises 61, 62–7
stroke
and atherosclerosis 2, 47
and cholesterol 22
and ethnic background 2
and exercise 59
risk factors 2, 9–13, 17, 27, 47
and sleep apnoea 49
sugar see carbohydrates
sumac-roasted chicken with beetroot &
almond salad 189
sweet chilli mayonnaise 224
sweet corn
. . . tinned 28
sweet corn & potato rösti 155
sweet potato
curried sweet potato cakes 208
roast lamb with sweet potato 236
swim, the 85

T
tabouli 223
tabouli & chickpea salad 203
tahini dressing 203
talk test 12, 71
tea 119
textured vegetable protein (TVP) 112
Thai beef kebabs 192
Thai green fish curry 211
thyme & lemon lamb cutlets with
zucchini & chickpea salad 230
Tick foods 25, 28, 119
tomatoes
. . . tinned 28
chargrilled steak sandwiches with
tomato relish 232
lamb & spinach meatballs with spicy
tomato sauce 197
pita bread, tomato & tuna salad 164
pizza with tomato, artichoke &
mushrooms 163
prawn & tomato soup with
mussels 180
tomato & herb salad 199
tomato & oregano cannelloni 206
tomato bruschetta 251
Total Wellbeing Diet 2, 116
training heart rate (THR) 69–71, 72
trans fats 24–5, 119

triceps
    dip 82
    exercises 81–2
    stretch 66
triglycerides 254, 265
    and blood glucose 31
    and blood pressure 10, 265
    and cardiovascular disease 25
    causes of high levels 25–6
    and cholesterol 10, 265
    effect of CLIP 3, 26, 97, 103, 115
    and CLIP dinner options 115, 261
    and heart attack 2
    lowering 25–6
    and long-chain omega-3 fatty acids
      93
    measurement 10, 22
    and stroke 2
    and wholegrain foods 97
trout *see* fish
tuna
    . . . tinned 28
    tuna, corn & coriander patties 224
    tuna pasta bake 215
turkey 117
TVP *see* textured vegetable protein
    (TVP)
type 2 diabetes
    and abdominal fat 17
    and blood glucose 31–3
    and blood-pressure medication 30
    and cardiovascular disease 2, 12,
      22, 48
    causes 31–2
    effects 32
    and erectile dysfunction 39, 40
    and exercise 32, 34, 59, 70
    and heart attack 2
    medication 32–3
    and sleep 49
    and stress 44, 48
    and stroke 2
    and triglyceride levels 31, 32
    and weight loss 31, 32
    and wholegrain foods 97

U

unsaturated fats 41, 96, 112, 116, 119,
    253
upper-arm stretch 65
upper-back exercises 80

upper-back stretch 64
upper-body exercises 74, 77–83
upper-body stretches 64–7
upper-leg exercises 87–8
upright row 80

V

vegetable moussaka 176
vegetable samosa parcels 208
vegetable suggestions 199
vegetables
    on CLIP 3, 29, 107, 113, 114, 117
    and erectile dysfunction 41
    fibre content 20, 95
    on Free Lists 105
    heart-protective food 108
    recommended intake 29
    salt content 28
    and weight loss 52
vegetarians and CLIP 110–12, 118–19
vegie burger with herb aïoli 158
vinaigrette
    for chicken, snow pea & pumpkin
      salad 164
    lemon 164, 184

W

waist circumference
    and cardiovascular disease 11
    and health 11
    measurement 11, 18
walking program 68–72, 259; *see also*
    aerobic walking
warm-up before exercise 61
water tablets 30
weight 10–11
    and exercise 59
    and sexual problems 39
    and sleep 49, 50
weight loss
    and blood pressure 27
    and cardiovascular disease 2, 17
    and cholesterol 108–9
    effect of CLIP 3
    and exercise 34, 36
    and HDL cholesterol 24, 25
    for men 18
    motivation for 51–5
    rapidity 18
    setting goals 17–18, 51–5
    with sex 39

strategies 20–21
    for women 18
wholegrain cereals 28
    and cardiovascular disease 97
    on CLIP 2, 97–8, 106
    fibre content 20, 97–8
    heart-protective food 108
    and type 2 diabetes 97
    types 97
wholemeal lemon crepes with
    raspberries 246
winter lamb casserole 194

Y

yoghurt
    . . . on CLIP 104, 117
    . . . plant-sterol-enriched 104
    chargrilled salmon with lentils,
      spinach & yoghurt 211
    cumin yoghurt 178
    Indian pork curry with minted
      yoghurt & basmati rice 228
    lemon yoghurt dressing 163, 216
    poached stone fruit with
      yoghurt 240
    spicy carrot & yoghurt dip 173

Z

zucchini
    chargrilled beef with zucchini, pine
      nuts & spinach 178
    prawn & salmon risotto with lemon
      & zucchini 218
    thyme & lemon lamb cutlets with
      zucchini & chickpea salad 230
    zucchini & chickpea salad 230
    zucchini & feta soup 236
    zucchini & pea fritters with smoked
      salmon & herbs 163